ACNE
AN ACTUAL
CURE

ACNE AN ACTUAL CURE

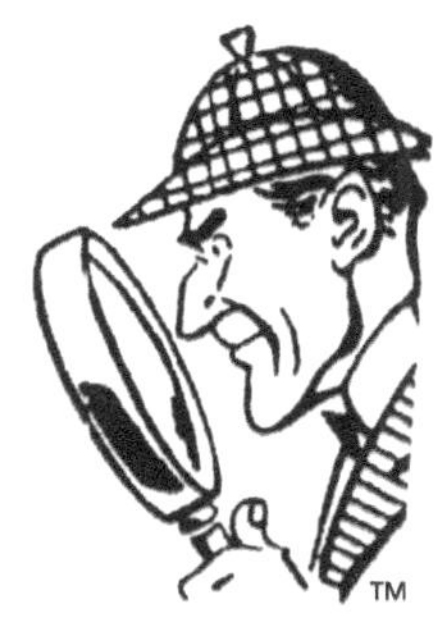

Who gets cured
Who doesn't
and why

Alfred V. Zamm, M.D.

DR. ZAMM'S MEDICAL MYSTERIES SERIES—VOL. 7 ED. 1

ISBN: 9798344097305

*With much appreciation to Judith Kistler
for her help and skill in the preparation and
editorialization of this book*

and to

*Margaret Cirillo, Librarian,
for her help in the forensic process of
tracking down medical clues.*

Disclaimer

This book is designed for informational purposes only. It is not a medical prescription, it is not medical advice, nor is it a suggestion for individual medical care. Medical care to an individual should only be provided by a licensed medical physician to a person who is enrolled with that physician in a formal physician-patient relationship.

In regard to any statement in this book, you are advised to discuss it with the medical practitioner with whom you are formally enrolled and not to take anything or do anything—health wise—without first receiving medical advice from your personal physician about your personal medical needs, as the material herein is provided for information only and not as medical advice. Since we are all the same and yet different, "one size" will not fit all: some of the observations and statements in this book will apply to—and be effective for—some individuals and yet not apply to or be effective for other individuals.

Table of Contents

Introduction

Let's approach your acne problem as a crime scene: The hidden *criminal* is the mechanism that is causing your acne (the *crime*). The *victim* is you, an innocent party.

I am a board-certified dermatologist with 60 years of experience in this capacity. During these 60 years, I have never prescribed topical or systemic antibiotics, isotretinoin (sold under the brand names of Accutane and others), hormones, or any other reputed "anti-acne" medicaments—except for the first few years of my medical practice, when I was a young and inexperienced dermatologist and didn't yet know the scientific information that I'm about to share with you.

I want to emphasize now and right up front: **Acne is not a disease**; it is a localized **symptom** of an underlying systemic disease, and that disease not only produces acne but also other life-altering symptoms that are taking away from the quality of your life. For a list of these other symptoms, see the back of this book for the listing entitled "Common Complaints...." But, in an attempt to give you some information now, a few possible other symptoms (but **not necessarily always present**) are: chronic fatigue, inability to concentrate, poor school grades, joint pains, and more, much more.

I will be your tour guide, and together we will go on an adventure of discovery and investigate the medical mystery of why you have acne (and uncover more about your health than you can imagine).

Bon voyage,
Alfred V. Zamm, M.D.

The approach you will learn in this book will not cure certain conditions by itself, although it may improve them. In addition to me you will need a specialist in that additional disorder. These other diseases are:

1. Acne due to a hormonal disturbance called polycystic ovary syndrome); this occurs only in women; you will need a hormone specialist (an endocrinologist);
2. Some cases of anemia (particularly in women); you will need an expert in blood diseases (a hematologist), since not all cases of anemia are simply due to iron deficiency. An expanded explanation of this anemia connection is beyond the scope of this treatise.
3. The side effects of lithium therapy. Even though acne can be associated with lithium therapy, the approach in this book can be very helpful).

Although it is very unorthodox, I am going to provide the following information within the introduction because that's where it conceptually belongs. I know my editor wouldn't permit this, so please don't tell her.

The following is an excerpt, one of the 24 essays in my book *Medical Secrets I Never Told You*. I'm including it here because it is the quickest way for you to grasp the entirety of what you're about to experience.

Essay 7

THE CASE OF THE SUICIDAL SOPHOMORE

I became suspicious the moment Evelyn C, a 20-year-old former college student, entered the examining room. She was seeing me professionally for the first time because of her facial blemishes (acne) of two years' duration. She looked extremely fatigued and depressed—an appearance way out of proportion to the relatively minor nature of her facial blemishes.

After we'd talked for a while, Evelyn revealed that, in addition to her blemishes, for the last two years she had been suffering from fatigue, depression, and had thoughts of suicide. This interesting relationship—all of her symptoms starting at the same time—was an intriguing clue that might be a clue that would unlock another medical mystery.

Evelyn told me that she had seen a variety of health practitioners and that, despite all the lotions, salves, and antibiotic pills prescribed for her, her acne remained stubbornly unresponsive. I explained to Evelyn that acne is an "inside problem" and that putting medicines on the outside won't fix what has gone wrong on the inside, even if some slight improvement does occur. Moreover, taking an antibiotic by mouth does not make the patient be better but only look better. And this superficial cosmetic effect soon disappears when the antibiotic is stopped. Unfortunately, the patient afterwards is left with two problems: The original acne problem and the side effects from taking antibiotics on a long-term basis. These side effects can include: the overgrowth of yeast in the gastrointestinal tract, the development of allergy to yeast and related fungi as a result of this increased yeast exposure, yeast infections, and the development of resistant strains of bacteria, not to mention the side effects of the drug itself. All of these disadvantages and yet no real cure for all of the trouble and expense of taking antibiotics day after day and, in some cases, year after year.

I told Evelyn that the older the patient is who has acne, the greater is the chance that there's some underlying internal cause for it. Acne often is the surface messenger that announces the presence of a deeper medical problem. Medical problems sometimes associated with acne are anemia and hormonal disturbances. Evelyn was tested and she didn't have these medical problems.

When all other possible causes for acne have been explored, the doctor must then consider a food allergy. In my experience, food allergy is the most common cause of acne in such resistant cases. I proceeded to outline a program of "medical sleuthing" for Evelyn. She was shown how to keep a detailed daily diary of everything she ate and to note any changes in her acne from day to day. I also asked her to save the labels from every manufactured food she ate so that we would both know the actual contents of the foods that she was eating. Different foods were alternatively omitted and added back into her diet to see what effect these foods would have on her symptoms. Very soon a pattern emerged: Evelyn ate spaghetti sauce, ketchup, and pizza addictively. Almost every meal had something made from tomato in it. She would even use ketchup on whatever she ate for breakfast—sometimes, she confessed, she even put it on corn flakes! Addictive eating of a particular single food is often a sign of food allergy. There was a similar but lesser addictive pattern relating to beef. Both of these foods were removed from her diet and improvement occurred over a four-week period. To prove to both of us that these foods were actually causing her acne, Evelyn was asked to try these omitted foods. Her acne returned. It should be understood that these foods are not harmful; it's just that Evelyn's body "made a mistake" and reacted allergically to these harmless substances.

All was going well; Evelyn carefully stayed on her diet, not eating beef or tomato, when inexplicably her acne, fatigue, and depression returned. Further investigation—again by having her record everything she ate—revealed that she was now eating eggplant. Often when a patient is allergic to one member of a food family, that patient can also be allergic to some or all of the other members of that food family. This is called cross-reactivity. Not surprisingly, eggplant belongs to the tomato family; it is sort of a "giant tomato". Evelyn was investigated and was not found to be allergic to potato, red or green pepper, or other members of this family. When she stopped eating eggplant, her symptoms again disappeared - this time for good.

What is particularly interesting about Evelyn's story is that her tomato allergy not only produced acne, but it also produced depression, difficulty concentrating, fatigue, and confusion—**all central nervous system symptoms**. Evelyn later told me that she had left college because she couldn't concentrate, which resulted in her not being able to keep up with the work. Once these foods were completely eliminated from her diet, her mental clarity returned, the other mental symptoms disappeared, and she decided to return to college.

What is the connection between acne, fatigue, depression, confusion, inability to concentrate, and food allergy? The allergic process, when it occurs, does not just occur in one organ alone; it is a systemic process that occurs throughout the entire body. And any organ in the body can be affected. However, symptoms may show up more in one area than another. Evelyn's beef allergy only gave her acne. But her tomato allergy involved her brain as well as her skin.

Neurological allergy and food allergy: When allergy symptoms occur in the skin, we call it a "rash". When they occur in the nose, we say the patient has "rhinitis or hay fever". When the symptoms are in the lungs, we call it "asthma". What should one call a "rash" (inflammation) of the brain? It's called brain dysfunction. Examples of brain dysfunction that often have a partial allergic component (together with a genetic component) are: Attention Deficit Disorder Syndrome (can't focus the mind) and Hyperkinetic Syndrome (can't focus the mind and disruptively active). Children who have either of these two conditions do not do well in school. These children grow up to become adults who do not do well in life. These individuals can often (not always) be helped by a simple program similar to the one that Evelyn followed. A more common but less successful method of dealing with these neurological problems is symptomatic therapy by taking medication, often with many undesirable side effects and, of course, no cure.

Another term for this type of allergy is "neurological allergy"—a subject that has received more attention in the last 20 years. Unfortunately, it is not commonly thought of and, hence, not often diagnosed. This is a subject of great importance and occurs more commonly than most people realize. In fact, the most common symptom of allergy is not a runny nose or asthma but fatigue, another symptom of neurological allergy. Evelyn was lucky that she had a skin problem that prompted her to seek medical attention. However, many patients don't show any outward manifestations of allergy—no rash, no itching—and yet suffer from the same kind of mental symptoms that Evelyn had. These patients almost never connect their mental suffering with a neurological allergic cause, and often they endure a lifetime of mental suffering—needlessly.

With any type of mental dysfunction, a possible physical reason for the mental symptoms should always be considered. If the subject of physical causes of mental disturbance has not been brought up by the health practitioner, it should be proposed by the patient. Neurological allergy commonly occurs and is just one of many physical conditions that cause mental dysfunction. Paradoxically it is the one that is most often overlooked and yet is the easiest to treat: stop eating (or breathing) the troublesome substance.

References

Sulzberger MB, Baer RL: Acne vulgaris and its management: A guide for the practitioner, in Sulzberger MB and Baer, RL (eds): *The 1949 YearBook of Dermatology and Syphilology*. Chicago, The Year Book Publishers, 1950, pp 9-39.

Zamm AV: Chronic urticaria: The role of food allergy. *Cutis*. 11:670-673, 1973.

Speer F: *Allergy of the Nervous System*. Springfield, Charles C. Thomas, 1970.

Chapter 1

HOW TO BE A MEDICAL DETECTIVE—THE OVERALL PLAN

We will divide what is to be an instructional manual into two parts (two plans):

- **Plan A**: The easier way, the statistical way: betting the favorite
- **Plan B:** If Plan A is not enough, we use Plan B, a more comprehensive way to uncover the criminal that is committing the crime of food allergy.

We will use Plan B to solve difficult problems because it *eliminates* the criminal's trick of using invisibility ("masking") to elude capture (*vide infra*). Plan B is used when food allergy is a suspected diagnosis, but no specific allergenic food comes to mind and any food can turn out to be allergenic. **This is in contrast to Plan A, when only one food**

is under suspicion (as is cow's milk in Plan A *vide infra*). Fear not, dear reader: enjoy the adventure, have some fun; all of these interesting details will be explained to you, and you too can achieve the rank of medical detective.

Chapter 2

PLAN A: THE DETAILS

As a result of my 60 years of clinical experience as a board-certified specialist in dermatology, I found **the most common allergenic food** to be **cow's milk (including all of its products—whey, milk solids, casein, cheese, etc.**). It is allergenic by itself or mixed in with other foods. *NB* Cow's milk is not poisonous or dangerous if you're not allergic to it. But if you are allergic to it (as with any other allergenic substance) it is dangerous and allergenically destructive via the chronic, persistent inflammation (not infection) it engenders.

Here are three easily recognized but often overlooked clues that have helped me to suspect that **cow's milk allergy** was the criminal—*remember*, you can have cow's milk allergy and still not have any **recognizable** symptoms and yet structure in your body can still be a target of cow's milk allergy. (For a list of other possible symptoms—clues to the existence of cow's milk acting as an allergen—see "Common Complaints" [Appendix I]).

Clues:

1. A childhood history of ear infections (this is the best clue to the existence of cow's milk allergy—nearly 100% accurate).
2. A history of asthma (a frequently valid clue but not one exclusive to the existence of cow's milk allergy— other allergens can cause asthma). If the asthma started in childhood, the accuracy of cow's milk allergy being a criminal approaches 100%.
3. A history of acne (again, a valid clue but not exclusive to cow's milk allergy, as there are other causes of acne—other food allergies and

non-allergenic causes); however, if the acne is **severe** (Grade III or Grade IV), the likelihood of cow's milk allergy being at least one cause of the patient's acne approaches 100%).

Fatigue is the most common symptom of any kind of allergy (food, inhalants, etc.); it is the best clue to watch for when eating a food as a test for allergenicity. Yes, I agree—vague and sometimes difficult to discern, but still the best and the most consistently accurate diagnostic clue. *NB:* I have frequently witnessed previously undetected food allergy to be a cause of a patient's chronic and unexplained fatigue—most often cow's milk allergy.

Masking: what is it and why is it important? The best method for detecting a food allergy is also the simplest: **eat the suspected food after masking (*vide infra*) is removed and watch for symptoms.**

- **Masking: the overview:**
  If you remember this one phrase, this maxim will help you remember how masking works: "The food that makes you feel better now makes you feel worse later." The "feeling better" is the patient's immediate and connected pleasurable perception of masking at the time of eating the food. The feeling worse occurs later, when this connection may not be made by the victim. (We are indeed in an Alice-in-Wonderland world of allergy inhabited by a clever criminal.)

  The trick to understanding masking is **not** to think of food allergy as a linear process of "you eat the allergenic food every day and then you are provoked every time you eat it, thus making you feel worse every time you eat it." That's **not** the way masking and this aspect of the world of allergy works.

- **<u>Masking: the details in an outline form:</u>**

(1) You would think that eating the food and the provocation would occur about the same time, but that may not be the case in this commonly occurring form of allergy if the person is already allergic to the responsible food, ***eats it frequently*** and ***perhaps every day*** or multiple times in a day, and has antibodies and other allergenic substances against that particular food.

(2) **A person who constantly eats the allergenic food will always have some of that food or derivatives of that food present internally**.

(3) As a result of the repetitive exposure to the responsible food, allergy develops to that food.

(4) Because of the frequent exposure to that allergenic food, the ***magnitude*** of the allergic response is

never maximum in severity and never minimum in severity and the ***allergic symptoms are low-level and always present*** because the antibodies and other allergenic modalities against the food are continually being used up as well as being generated. The patient always lives under a pall of low-level allergic symptoms and accepts this burden of constant low-level allergic symptoms as "normal," i.e., "normal" constant fatigue, "normal" constant brain fog, "normal" constant stiff muscles, "normal" constant joint pain, etc.—"normal" as in symptoms always being present ("normally" being sick) but "not normal" in the sense of being healthy. See "Common Complaints" in the Appendix for a list of more symptoms of food allergy—symptoms that the victim may not associate with allergy as a cause.

(5) If a person eats an allergenic food that produces undesirable allergic symptoms, why keep eating the food?

(6) As previously stated, the victim eats the allergenic food often and *addictively* because: a) **the time of eating and b) the time that symptoms occur** are separated, often by hours, a part of a day, an entire day, or the next day; hence, the victim doesn't connect the *cause* (the eating of the allergenic food) with the **effect** (the symptoms that occur later). These symptoms (pleasure and the uncomfortable state of illness) are conceptually opposite, and no rational and untrained person would usually connect them.

(7) The victim connects the food to the ***pleasure*** that occurs ***when*** the food is eaten and not to the ***discomfort*** that gradually occurs ***later***. The victim likes eating the food and will often say that it's a favorite food (the criminal is clever).

(8) The nature of the ***undesirable symptoms*** can be vague, elusive, and ***low-level***; some examples were just mentioned: fatigue, brain fog, a low level of muscular "stiffness" (myalgia), or a low level of joint pains (arthralgia), head-aches, mental depression and more (see Common Complaints in Appendix I)

(9) **In summary: A victim having this type of food allergy may never realize that the food—perhaps a favorite food, maybe one that is eaten frequently—is the crimi-nal.** The victim may constantly and

addictively eat the food and live in a mad allergenic rollercoaster world of contrasting overlapping cycles of feeling better, with pleasure, and feeling worse, with undesirable symptoms—a phantasmagorical Alice-in-Wonderland world of allergy having no perceptible logic. Yes, you may be thinking all of this sounds like alcoholism (and other addictions), and you are right. The mechanism that drives addiction has a masking component. Alcoholics are almost always allergic to one or more of the ingredients in what they are pleasurably and addictively imbibing.

Unmasking and testing—the details:

A. Unmasking
    It's only when the consumption of the allergenic food is **stopped for**

five days that the masking process is eliminated. At that point:

1. Eating the food (as a test) will reveal the truth of whether the food is allergenic or not.
2. Allergic symptoms will be revealed in a pristine manner without the symptom-mitigating process of masking.
3. The provoked symptoms will be revealed in a ***greater*** magnitude because the masking of the allergenic food was eliminated.
4. Think of this as five days of ***accumulated potential and uninstigated reaction*** (the accumulation of unused provocative inflammatory bodily chemicals).
5. I think of this as five "firecrackers" of accumulated potential explosion going off all at once rather than being spread out and going off a little at a time (one firecracker each day over five days).

B. Testing

This type of provocative food test-ing, where masking has been elimi-nated, is:

1. More accurate than blood or skin tests for food allergy NOTE: This test **reaction** will include by the body not only IgE antibod-ies (reagin) **but non-reagin sub-stances that are not testable in a doctor's office—all combine** to produce a now powerful and clin-ically discernible, pristine explo-sive allergic reaction unaffected by the potentially obscuring and mitigating masking process. (Reference: Coca AF: Familial Non-Reagin Food-Allergy. Lyle Stuart. Secaucus NJ 4th ed. August 1982.)

2. Quick

3. At no cost

4. Convenient—the patients can do it all by themselves and at home.

5. Educational: it imparts an understanding of masking and how to test for food allergy that empowers patients to be their own medical detectives—a skill that will help them for the rest of their lives. I think of this in terms of the proverb, "Give a man a fish and he will eat for a day; teach him how to fish and he will eat for the rest of his life."

<u>A comment on masking</u>:

A **more technical** explanation of why there is a temporary and counterintuitive **reduction** of clinical symptoms and, additionally, an **associated pleasurable response** during the masking process involves antibodies, prostaglandins, cytokines, interleukins, T-cells, B-cells, cyclical food allergy and, most importantly, neurotransmitters, is beyond the scope of this essay. (Trust me; let's let all of that go and get back to the narrative of our adventure; we will both be better off for it).

<u>Testing for inhalant allergies—an entirely different story</u>.

> N.B: In contrast to **food allergy,** objective skin and blood **tests** for ***inhalant* allergy** due to pollens, molds, house dust, etc., involve antibodies and ***are*** accurate.

<u>Anaphylaxis (the most blatant example of "immediate hypersensitivity"):</u>
All of this brings to mind a type of food allergy that masking ***does not involve***: the notorious and deadly peanut allergy, where a person who has this type of response eats a peanut and then collapses with multiple symptoms, such as shortness of breath, muscle spasm, itching, and more, and possibly death. These patients have a very high blood level of an antibody called IgE. IgE ***is*** measurable by a blood test.

<u>**How to test for any food allergy (in this case, cow's milk):**</u>

1. The patient completely stops eating cow's milk and all cow's milk products for five days (the five-day mandatory ***clearing period*** to eliminate the masking effect).

   We use a five-day elimination period for this single food, which is longer than Dr. Randolph's two-day elimination period, because our patient is not existing only on distilled water, as was the case with Dr. Randolph's patients (*vide infra*).

2. The patient then ***carefully*** tries cow's milk (whole milk, not skim) and observes for provoked symptoms such as ***fatigue, asthma, itching, other***. For other possible symptoms of allergenic provocation, see "Common Complaints," in the Appendix.

3. When the patient carefully tests a food by ingesting it, the patient ***tries***

only a little bit at the beginning of the testing process. In the case of cow's milk, an ounce—and then *waits an hour* to proceed, as the symptoms will be exaggerated and could be severe, because the protective effect of masking has been removed by having stopped the food for five days. If no provocation occurs, the patient then tries two ounces of cow's milk; if no reaction occurs, the patient probably is not allergic to cow's milk. *It should be noted that a clinically observable reaction may occur later—hours later or even the next day*. This is called a *delayed reaction* in contrast to an *immediate reaction*. In the case of a delayed reaction, and not to miss it, **don't** test any other food before noon of the **following day**. If the patient still has not displayed a reaction by 12:00 noon of the following day, you can assume in most cases that all is well, and you can proceed to testing the next food *as would happen when utilizing Plan B* (*vide infra*). Remember not to overlook fatigue as a symptom—common to occur, easy to miss. If the patient is found to be allergic to cow's milk, cow's milk must be avoided 100% in all forms, all the time, and for life.

The following comments refer only to Plan B (vide infra):

You must wait until you are feeling reasonably better from your reaction before you can go on and test the next food on your list. It may take one day or longer for the reaction to pass. Any food you're not sure about should be avoided and can be tested later. If you continue to eat a food that you're not sure about, the results of the next series of tests will not be clear and you will not know which food is inducing your symptoms.

<u>**It's a myth that cow's milk is
an essential nutrient:**</u>

The **only** foods that are essential for humans are the following five elemental foods (in addition to water, of course):

1. *Protein*
2. **Fats**
3. **Carbohydrates**
4. **Vitamins**
5. **Minerals**

<u>**There is nothing special about cow's milk except the following:**</u>

1. It is the bodily secretion of a barn animal intended for baby cows;
2. It has a very high potential for allergenicity in humans;
3. It is not an essential food (vida supra);
4. It is not essential for human babies;
5. What is essential for human babies?
    a. The best choice: Mother's breast milk

b. The next best choice: Substitute one of the many scientifically formulated **non-cow's milk** babies' milk substitutes that are commercially available.

A comment on vitamin D:

There is no significant amount of vitamin D in cow's milk; it is added to the cow's milk by the milk company. You can optimally meet your nutritional requirement yourself by taking vitamin D_3, 2,000 iu per day.

A comment on calcium

Calcium is not unique to cow's milk. For example, there is twice as much calcium weight-for-weight in soybeans as compared with cow's milk. That's how the cow gets the calcium it nutritionally needs and then puts some of it into the milk that you buy—it eats soybeans in the meal that it is fed.

There is plenty of calcium in vegetable "milks" such as soybean "milk", rice "milk," almond "milk," oat "milk," etc. Nutritionally biochemically identical Vitamin D and calcium are added to these "milks" in adequate amounts by the manufacturer.

The problem with Plan A is that it is limited to one food, cow's milk; if a patient has more food allergies, then Plan B will have to be used.

While we're on the subject of cow's milk allergy, here are some comments and scientific references on cow's milk allergy that illustrate how widespread, pernicious, and unrecognized by the general public cow's milk allergy is. This technical information is only a sample of what is available in the medical literature on this subject and is provided for those readers who are curious and intrepid and for my physician colleagues.

1. Davies DF, Johnson AP, Rees BW, et al: Food antibodies and myocardial

infarction. *Lancet* 1974 May 25;1(7865): 1012-4 PMID: 4133698 [PubMed-indexed for MEDLINE]

2. Fourier E: Allergy to cow's milk. *Allerg Immunol* (Paris). 1997 Apr;29(4):108-10. PMID: 9213419

3. Law-Chin-Yung L, Freed DL: Nephrotic syndrome due to milk allergy. *Lancet*. 1977 May 14;1(8020):1056. PMID: 67516. Doi: 10.1016/s0140-6736(77)91291-0.

4. De Sousa JS, Rosa FC, Baptista A, et al: Cow's milk protein sensitivity: a possible cause of nephrotic syndrome in early infancy. *J Pediatr Gastroenterol Nutr.* 1995 Aug;21(2):235-7. PMID: 7472914. DOI: 10.1097/00005176-199508000-0019.

5. Bahna SL: Control of milk allergy: A challenge for physicians, mothers and industry. *Annals of Allergy* Vol 41, No 1, July 1978

6. Clein NW: Cow's milk allergy in infants. *Ann. Allergy*, 9:195, 1951.

7. Dees SC: Allergy to cow's milk. *Pediat Clin N Amer*, 6:881, 1959.

8. Collins-Williams C: Cow's milk allergy in infants and children. Int. Arch. Allergy, 20:38, 1962.

9. Truelove SC: Ulcerative colitis provoked by milk. *Brit Med J*, 1:154, 1962.

10. Goldman AS, Anderson Jr, DWSellers, WA, et al: Milk allergy 1. Oral Challenge with Milk and Isolated Milk Proteins in Allergic Children. *Pediatrics* Vol 32, No 3, September 1963.

11. Debiec H, Lefeu F, Kemper M, et al: Early-Childhood Membranous Neuropathy Due to Cationic Bovine Serum Albumin. *N Engl J Med* 2011; 364:2101-10 2011

12. Gerrard JW: Familial Recurrent Rhinorrhea and Bronchitis Due to Cow's Milk *JAMA* 1966 Nov 7; Vol 198, No 6; 137-

13. Eggermont E: Cow's milk protein allergy. PMID: 69738350

Dear Reader, if you don't have the time to read or the facilities to obtain the above references and can obtain only one reference, the following book by Professor Frank Oski, M.D., is the one to read: *Don't Drink Your Milk* 3rd edition, published by Teach Services 2013. Professor Oski was Director of Pediatrics at Johns Hopkins University School of Medicine and also was Physician-in-Chief at the Johns Hopkins Children's Center.

This book is a unique, informative, and understandable contribution to the subject of the surprising and potentially perilous nature of cow's milk. The contents will surprise you.

Chapter 3

PLAN B: THE DETAILS

et's say the patient tried Plan A and either it didn't work or it didn't work well enough because there were other additional suspected allergic foods—in either case, the investigator decides to move on to Plan B.

Why I developed Plan B and what is its history?

Back in the late 1950's there was a small group of physicians (M.D.'s), who were all board certified in various medical specialties. Some were professors in medical schools, some were Chairmen of departments in hospitals, and all members had a strong interest in food allergy—as well as other medical interests.

This group was so interesting and academically productive that it rapidly grew, drawing physicians from all over the world. They called themselves The Human Ecology Society (later it morphed into its current name, The American Academy of Environmental Medicine). I was fortunate to have become a member of this group.

We held annual meetings drawing fine lecturers from all over the world. When we weren't at these meetings, we were visiting at each other's offices to see firsthand "what's new." When we couldn't do that, we were on the phone, sharing the latest ideas. The leader of our obsessed band of physicians was a board-certified internist, Theron Randolph, M.D. Among his many other achievements, Dr. Randolph developed a method of detecting elusive food allergies. His method was, briefly stated:

1. He admitted the patient to a specially designed **hospital unit** where the environment was controlled and pure in every way.
2. He placed the patient on a "diet" of **only** pure distilled water for two

days (thereby eliminating masking)—yes I did say "only" and we were obsessed).

3. He would add insecticide-free (organic) test foods back into the patient's diet one each day and be able to observe for now unmasked pristine allergic reactions.

I agree, this method was extreme and was difficult for the patient, for the physician, and for the hospital—"obsessed" is probably an understatement—but it worked. It worked when all other methods and other doctors had failed; Dr. Randolph cured many "incurable" patients. He was an inspiration to me—and to all of us. Oscar Wilde, the clever literary epigrammist of another era knew what it took to be successful when he quipped, "Nothing succeeds like excess." Dr. Randolph was his acolyte.

Productive as Dr. Randolph's method was, I had to find a modification of his method that an everyday patient might be willing to endure for at least a brief period, and at home.

The following Plan B's methods and patient instructions are my modification of Dr. Randolph's method—it has helped many patients to uncover their hidden food allergies (and to become good medical detectives).

Dear Reader, in this section you will be provided with the specific information you need to do Plan B. An overview of this is:

1. You will be using a defined diet to eliminate the masking effect. These foods are not usually allergenic and have a low occurrence in most diets.
2. After masking has been removed by the elimination diet, as previously explained, you will be adding foods back **one at a time.**
3. **If you are known to be intolerant to any of the suggested foods, delete that food from this initial diet designed to eliminate masking.**

THE DIET TO ELIMINATE MASKING

Only the following foods are to be eaten. **No other foods may be substituted**, however similar they may appear.

When in doubt, consult the list below. **If it's not on the list, don't eat it!** It is **not** necessary to eat **all** of the foods, but try to eat as many as possible, as this will be very helpful later in the investigation. Eat whatever you like from the foods on this list. For the duration of the test, you cannot eat in restaurants or at a friend's house. If you customarily eat some meals away from home, you must bring your foods with you. You will find plastic bags and vacuum bottles of great help in accomplishing your goal.

Food choices	Footnotes
Duck	
Shrimp	
Turkey	6
Asparagus	1, 2
Avocado	
Broccoli	1, 2
Brussels Sprouts	1, 2
Cabbage	1, 2
Cauliflower	1,2
Celery	2
Spinach	1, 2
Safflower Oil	7
Millet	
Rice	5
Sweet Potato	1, 2
Yam	1, 2
Salt	4
Water	3

All foods (except avocado) should be **cooked**. These items should be obtained fresh or frozen, if available—<u>not canned</u>.

Use frozen only if fresh is not in season. If frozen is used, you will not be able to wash the vegetables in detergent, as discussed within.

1. To reduce exposure to insecticide contamination of these foods, wash them as instructed below.
2. Do **NOT** drink chlorinated water. If the source of your drinking water is chlorinated, one of the following substitutions is permissible (listed in order of preference): 1) commercially purchased bottled water; 2) tap water boiled for a minute to drive off the chlorine and cooled. The source of the water should be mentioned in your diet record. Do NOT drink water from a water softener. Do **NOT** drink water having a "sulfur" taste (hydrogen sulfide).

3. Ordinary shaker salt may be used. Avoid iodized salt. Iodized salt is not only permissible, but it is desirable and may be resumed after the investigation.
4. Use only brown rice. Do **NOT** use rice cakes.
5. Turkey may be purchased fresh or frozen; however, it must be a whole turkey and **not** the prebasted variety. It **cannot** be turkey parts, turkey loaf, turkey roll, smoked or processed in any way.
6. Safflower oil should be purchased in a **glass bottle** and may be eaten cooked or raw.

Do not roast or bake in a **gas** oven. Do not use a cooktop-style potato baker with a **gas** stove (the gas is absorbed by the food and is harmful). Frying and boiling on a gas stove are **temporarily** permitted. Any form of cooking is permitted with an electric stove, electric cooktop, microwave, or any electric device. Do not charcoal broil. Do not use non-stick pans.

Do **not** chew gum or use candy, Life Savers, etc. Temporarily, do not use vitamins (vitamin C is OK) or ordinary toothpaste ("Tom's" natural **fennel** toothpaste without fluoride may be used and is available from natural food stores and online.

It is essential that you eat on this diet. Do not ty to deal with this diet by not eating or by reducing the amount of food you eat. If you do not do this, you will become excessively hungry, your bodily chemistry will not function properly, you will feel worse, and this initial portion of the investigation will be ruined. Use salt to taste. **If, despite this, fatigue occurs, replace potassium loss** with one tablet of potassium gluconate (approximately 610 mg = approximately 99 mg. of actual potassium) three times a day with food. Obtain potassium gluconate over the counter (no prescription necessary).

Eating pears (remove the skin) will work as a source of potassium; think of it as one pear = one tablet.

Every day you must eat <u>at least</u> three meals <u>plus</u> three snacks. Each meal and each snack must consist of a sampling of a protein, a vegetable, and a carbohydrate on this list:

- **Protein** (animal products) on the list
- **Vegetables** on the list
- A **carbohydrate** on the list (sweet potato, yam, millet, rice)

The only difference between a "meal" and a "snack" is the amount of food.

INSTRUCTIONS FOR
KEEPING A DIET RECORD

<u>Use the suggestions below</u> for keeping <u>a</u> <u>written record of everything you eat</u>. <u>Use a separate page for each day and date each page on top.</u>

Write down <u>all</u> the foods you are about to eat <u>before you eat them</u>. This will prevent you from accidentally eating a food that is not on the permitted diet and/or forgetting to write it down by <u>bringing it to your atten-tion before you eat it.</u>

1. <u>Keep a separate page as a record for each day</u>
2. <u>Each page should have the same heading</u>

<u>Day of the Week   Date   Page Number</u>

<u>These three items will appear identi-cally on the top of each page. Only the page numbers will change.</u>

3. <u>The layout of each day's record should include the following content:</u>
   a. The name of the food
   b. The time the food is eaten
   c. The location where the food is eaten
   d. Observations: any symptoms that are occurring at the time the food is being eaten (symptoms which may or may not be related to the food just eaten but may be related to location, i.e., the inhalation of ambient noxious materials or a delayed reaction from a previously ingested food—all this to be analyzed and decided upon after the entire experiment is over.)

NOTE: A symptom may occur at a time when no food has been eaten. The importance of recording these symptoms and when they occur cannot be overstated. The purpose of this is that a symptom may occur not at a time a food is being eaten and the cause of that symptom will be determined after all the information has been analyzed. (caused by a previously eaten food or a noxious substance had been inhaled).

HOW TO LESSEN YOUR EXPOSURE TO INSECTICIDES AND OTHER CHEMICALS ON FRUITS AND VEGETABLES

The relationship of cancer and other diseases to insecticides and other chemical residues in foods has been extensively discussed in the medical literature. Since we cannot stop eating, our only alternative is to lower these poisonous resides on the foods we eat.

The following method will help you to remove these externally applied poisonous substances from fruits and vegetables. Certain poisons pervade the inner portions of fruits and vegetables, and these will not wash out with this process. At least you will have done everything you can to lower the chances of having a problem from ingesting these externally applied chemicals.

METHOD: How to use three solutions of the same detergent:

(1) "Stock Solution"
(2) "Work Solution"
(3) "Washing Solution"

(1) THE "STOCK SOLUTION":

For the Stock Solution, use a liquid detergent sold for general kitchen use. It should not have any fragrance or color. The one I personally use is Seventh Generation brand of dishwashing liquid, and I specify <u>no color</u> and <u>no scent</u> liquid kitchen dishwashing detergent (since it comes two ways: with scent and without scent).

DO NOT USE THE "STOCK SOLUTION" FOR WASHING FRUITS AND VEGETABLES DIRECTLY FROM THE BOTTLE: IT MUST BE DILUTED. WASH FOODS ONLY WITH THE "WASHING SOLUTION" DESCRIBED BELOW.

(2) THE "WORK SOLUTION":

How to make the "work solution":

Pour a small amount of "stock solution" into an empty squeeze-type plastic bottle so that it fills 1/10 of the bottle. Then fill the rest of the bottle with tap water.

Shake the bottle to mix the water and stock solution. This is now the "work solution." This "work solution" is very convenient to use. Keep it handy to make the "washing solution" each time you prepare fruits and vegetables. You will use the "work solution" to make the "washing solution."

USE THE "WASHING SOLUTION" FOR WASHING FRUITS AND VEGETABLES

(3) THE "WASHING SOLUTION"

How to make and use the "washing solution":

Into a wide-mouthed bowl that holds approximately 2 quarts of tap water, put about one ounce of the "work solution"; fill the container with cold water until it is ¾ full. This will mix the "work solution" with fresh water and make copious suds. This mixture of "work solution" and water is the final "washing solution."

Place the prepared fruit or vegetable pieces into the container and swirl them in the "washing solution" for about a minute

How to prepare food for washing with the "washing solution":

Let's use broccoli as an example. The broccoli florets should be broken off so that small clumps of broccoli (rather than the whole head) can be washed in the "washing solution." Breaking the vegetable into small pieces allows the detergent to get into the crevices and exposes more of the insecticide-laden vegetable surface to the "washing solution" for cleansing. The more surface area that is exposed, the cleaner the vegetable will be.

Remove the washed fruit or vegetable pieces and put them into a colander. Rinse the pieces thoroughly in running tap water until all detergent residue is gone. Rinse generously; it is easy for a small amount of soap residue to remain. The food is now ready to be cooked. *Bon Appetit!*

Other vegetables that cannot be peeled should be similarly washed. Examples: cauliflower, spinach, string beans, etc.

Vegetables that absorb water rapidly because of their structure, such as celery, should be cleansed differently. Dip a vegetable brush in the above-described "washing solution" and scrub the celery. Then rinse with generous amounts of tap water. Do not soak these vegetables in the "work" or "washing" solutions, as they will absorb the soapy water very quickly and become inedible.

Some foods do not need to be washed in detergent:

It is not necessary to wash the inner leaves of those vegetables whose chemical residue-laden outer leaves can be removed. **Examples**: cabbage, Brussels sprouts.

Grapes and berries should be washed in the "**washing solution**" as above described, since the outer surfaces are eaten.

Fruits that can be peeled, the skins discarded, and whose interior pulp is eaten (bananas, oranges, apples, pears) do not require this treatment, since you will not be eating the skins. Don't try to wash apples and pears and then eat the skins. You will be more successful in avoid chemicals by peeling the skins and discarding them.

This is a quick summary of how to do it:

1. **The Stock Solution:** The original concentration of the unscented, uncolored dish detergent as it comes out of the commercial bottle.
2. **The Working Solution:** This is a **1:10 dilution** of the above Stock Solution in a plastic squeeze bottle.
3. **The Washing Solution:** One ounce of the Working Solution from the

squeeze bottle in Number 2 (above) into approximately two quarts of water in a wide-mouthed plastic bowl.

Dear Reader,
Now that you have been on this diet that eliminates the masking effect (yes, I know five days is long, but I'll accept four days if you must, and that will probably work). We're now ready to add foods back using the method in the discussion in the section following the discussion of milk allergy *vide supra.*

Certain foods are tricky because:

1. They are often found in a **manufactured form** and mixed with a commercially prepared food product; hence, you may not be aware of this connection.
2. A manufactured food (especially one that is heated) is not the same allergenically as a raw food. You will have to test the manufactured form of the

food as follows (remember to test one food at a time as previously outlined). You can test the raw (not manufactured form) of the food later.

a. **Corn**
   i. The commercially encountered form: corn oil, corn starch, corn sugar
   ii. The test form: cornmeal

b. **Cow's milk**
   i. The commercially encountered form: whole cow's milk, skimmed milk, whey, milk solids, casein
   ii. The test form: whole cow's milk (not skimmed)

c. **Wheat**
   i. The commercially encountered form: Bread and other baked goods.
   ii. The test form: whole wheat cereal (without additives such as malt, sugar, etc.).

d. **Egg**

   i. The commercially encountered form: egg whites, egg yolks

   ii. The test form: soft-boiled egg.

e. **Soybean**

   i. The commercially encountered form: soybean is encountered in many forms, often listed on ingredient labels, such as protein hydrolysate, soy oil

   ii. The test form: soy flour (obtainable in health food-type stores)

f. **Beef**

   i. The commercially encountered form: beef can be encountered in the form of gelatin ("Jello") and beef broth.

   ii. The test form: Steak, chopped meat, etc.

g. **Yeast**

Yeast is a complex subject; also see the Appendix.

i. Baker's yeast

    a. The commercially encountered form: baked foods.

    b. The test form: Buy baker's yeast in the grocery store (the dry form, as the other form may have cornstarch added to it). Just sprinkle 1/8 tsp. on some already tested and accepted food.

ii. Brewer's yeast

    a. The commercially available form: Vinegar, alcoholic beverages

    b. The test form: Brewer's yeast is obtainable in health food-type stores. Sprinkle 1/16 tsp. on accepted food.

Chapter 4

THE LEAKY GUT: WHAT IS IT, WHY IS IT, HOW IS IT?

So you think you have the answer. You found that you have food allergies and you have identified your specific allergenic foods; what are you going to do about it? Of course, you're going to stop eating the allergenic foods. But as perverse and counterintuitive as this may sound, there's more to dealing with food allergy than just stopping the consumption of allergenic foods.

A. Here are some thoughts on the mysteries of food allergy that have run through my mind:

1. Why do people develop food allergies?
2. How can they get rid of their food allergies?

3. How can they prevent the development of more food allergies?
   They developed food allergies once and they probably will keep doing it unless they discover the hidden reason why they did it in the first place.
4. Food allergy is the body's cry for help about a hidden problem; it is a plea in the form of symptoms that are coded messages (again, please see "Common Complaints" in the Appendix for a list of some of these coded-message symptoms). The ***symptoms of food allergy*** are clues to the existence of a secret pernicious driving process (the criminal) that is compromising the ***entire body,*** not just the part of the body that exhibits localized symptoms such as itching, coughing, etc.

B. Three essential facts that you need to hear about now but will make sense later:

1. People develop food allergies because of a failure to maintain an adequate electronic voltage on the secretory IgA molecule which rests on the absorptive gastrointestinal membrane.

2. Poisoning induces allergy: Poisoning interferes with the metabolic processes that supply electrons to the secretory IgA gatekeeper, thus lowering the voltage on the absorptive gastrointestinal membrane.

3. **Low** voltage results in a **greater transparency** of the gastrointestinal membrane and this leads to the so-called leaky gut, which sequentially leads to the development of food allergy. Hence, food allergy is an electronic process gone wrong.

I had to bring up this obscure information now in order to preserve continuity, and I've said too much already, so for now that's all I'm going to say on the subject because I don't want to interrupt the momentum of the narrative. A revelatory and expanded discussion of electronics, voltage, food allergy, and what you need to know on this subject can be found in Epilogues 2, 3, and 4. Fear not; it all will be explained, and it will be interesting, astounding, and fun.

There are environmental poisons that interfere with the metabolic mechanism that supplies electrons to the gatekeeper, and this reduces the voltage on the gastrointestinal membrane, thus leading to the development of food allergy.

The following is a list of common sources of poisoning that I have found to induce the development of allergy (***and the elimination of which I have found to mitigate or entirely eliminate existing allergies and prevent the development of new allergies***):

1. **<u>Poisoning from Mercury</u>**

   a. **<u>Exogenous sources of mercury</u>**:

      Large predatory fish such as tuna, swordfish, orange roughy, shark, tile fish, and **King** mackerel (other mackerel are OK), are significant dietary sources of mercury from nature. My dietary solution to the mercury-seafood problem is: I avoid eating large predatory fish and eat only low-mercury-containing fish like salmon, regular mackerel, small fish like sardines, and non-fish seafood (shrimp, crayfish, lobster).

      Another solution to the problem of mercury poisoning: I take selenium. The selenium atom proactively intercepts environmental poisonous heavy metals (including mercury) before they can combine with an enzyme and disable it. This protective combination is irrevocable; it permanently inactivates this poison, thus saving the enzyme from being disabled (for more about selenium, see Epilogue 1).

b. **<u>Endogenous sources of poisoning by mercury</u>:**

Poisoning from standard dental care (Yes, I did say "standard" as approved by the dental authorities). Mercury-containing dental fillings are an anachronistic concoction conceived in the early 1800s; it is an inheritance from the past, "grandfathered in" without any scientific proof of safety.

Chronic daily exposure to mercury from mercury-containing dental fillings—so-called "silver" dental fillings or amalgam dental fillings—is a source of daily poisoning. These "silver" dental fillings are deceptively called "silver fillings" but are actually 50%

mercury and only 30% silver and should be called "mercury fillings." (No one would buy them if the insidious poisonous nature of this mercury were revealed by the dentist to the unsuspecting patient—the customer that is about to become a victim.)

NB: Not only is mercury poisonous directly to metabolic processes, it also combines with the essential trace element selenium, thus depriving the body of valuable selenium. Selenium is a unique essential nutrient that the body incorporates into the defensive enzyme glutathione peroxidase (glutathione peroxidase defends against excessive endogenously derived oxidative substances). Selenium has many other functions in the body, and mercury will also deprive the body of these additional vital functions.

Selenium is protective against acquiring cancer. (See Epilogue 1)

It defies credulity that licensed dental professionals, the dental and medical professional organizations, the Food and Drug Administrations (both dental and medical divisions) allow the prescribing of mercury, a known poison (Mercury is number 80 in the Periodic Table, and by virtue of its atomic radius and number of electron shells it is incontrovertibly and scientifically a poison.). This is a gross abrogation of responsibility by all of these professional organizations acting in unison as a cabal of professional miscreants foisting a known toxic substance on a trusting public, a public that doesn't have the technical knowledge to defend itself, and telling them a poison is not a poison (a most egregious example of "gaslighting" on a massive and professional level).

In regard to these derelict professional organizations and the equally derelict government agencies, a proverb comes to mind: "if you see a crime being committed and you do nothing about it, you become a participant in that crime."

Now you are asking yourself, why don't these professional organizations and government agencies just recommend that dental mercury be taken off the market? My answer is: they can't. If they were to make that determination, it would be an admission that mercury is what it always has been: a poison. And then it becomes an admission of guilt, resulting in financial consequences that would be devastating for those that allowed this massive poisoning to take place— so they go on poisoning and ruining the lives of the vulnerable, trusting, unsuspecting innocent customers of the dentists who provide the mercury—merchants of death.

That other scientists feel the same way about mercury poisoning from "silver" amalgam dental fillings is demonstrated in this sample of the many peer-reviewed scientific references from the medical literature:

1. Eggleston DW: Effect of dental amalgam and nickel alloys on T-lymphocytes: Preliminary report. J. Prosthetic Dentistry, 1984; 51-617-23.

   Dear Reader, the above article is a very important one. Dr. Eggleston's research proves that mercury can depress T-cells. T-cells are like state troopers in that they defend against the "bad guys" (microorganisms, cancer). Anything that will depress the amount of T-cells in the body will lower the ability of the body to defend itself against infection, cancer, etc.—you get the point. The presence of mercury in the body pre-disposes the body to having diseases due to infections and cancer. It's not my opinion; Dr. Eggleston proved that mercury depresses T-cells. For my professional colleagues and those who are so inclined, I suggest you read the article. It's a wonderful piece of research.

2. Pleva J: Mercury poisoning from dental amalgam. J. Orthomol Psychiat. 1983; 12:184-93.

3. Koller, LD: Immunosuppression produced by lead, cadmium, and mercury. Am. J. Vet. Res. 1973; 34:1457-58.

4. Lawrence DA: Heavy metal modulation of lymphocyte activities. In vitro effects of heavy metals on primary humoral immune response. Toxicol. Appl. Pharmacol. 1981; 57:349-451.

5. Gilman AG, Rall TW, Niew AS, et al (eds): Goodman and Gilman's The Pharmacological Basis of

Therapeutics, 8th ed. New York, NY: Pergamon Press, 1990; 1598-1602.

6. Hahn LJ, Kloiber R, Vimy MJ, et al: Dental "silver" tooth fillings: a source of mercury exposure revealed by whole-body image scan and tissue analysis. The FASEB Journal. 1989; 3:2641-2646.

7. Hahn LJ, et al: Dental "silver" tooth fillings: a source of mercury exposure revealed by whole-body image scan and tissue analysis. The FASEB Journal. 1989; 3:2641-2646.

My solutions to a patient's problem with poisoning from their mercury-containing fillings are:

- Removal of these poisonous dental fillings by a dentist familiar with these matters (use a trusted dentist that does not prescribe these fillings);
- Take selenium (see Epilogue #1)

2. <u>Poisoning from root canals by the same cabal of professional miscreants</u>:

ROOT CANALS: another deception perpetrated on an unsuspecting public consists of more professionally prescribed poison, the insertion of root canals by dentists.

Root canals have at least three health problems:

1. They are very frequently (always?) infected, and hence a source of microbiologically derived cytotoxic and immune dysregulating substances.
2. They are endodontically executed using xenobiotic, cytotoxic, and often proprietary substances that are potentially immune dysregulating; and
3. There is not adequate scientific proof (double blind crossover studies) of the safety of the materials used in the "root canal" (endodontic) procedure.

Some samples of references from the peer-reviewed medical literature documenting that other scientists feel the same way about the danger of root canals:

1. Nagaoka S., Miyazaki Y., et al: Bacterial invasion into dentinal tubules of human vital and nonvital teeth. J Endod. 1995; Feb;21(2):70-3, PMID: 7714440.
2. Uchin, R.A.; Parris, L.: Antibacterial activity of endodontic medications after varying time intervals within the root canal. Oral Surg. 1963; 16:608-1
3. Tronstad L.: Yang, A.P.; Trope, M.; Barnett, F.; Hammond, B.: Controlled release of medicaments in endodontic therapy. Endod Dent Traumatol. 1985; 1:130-4.
4. Engstrom, B.; Spangbert, L.: Studies on root canal medicaments. 1. Cytotoxic effect of root canal antiseptics. Acid Odontol Scand. 1967; 25:77-84.

5. Spangbert, L.; Engstrom, B.: Studies on root canal medicaments. 11. Antimicrobial effect of root canal medicaments. Odontol Revy 1968; 2:187-95.

6. Moller, AJR: Microbial examination of root canals and peripical tissues of human teeth. Thesis. Odontol Tidskr (Special Issue) 1966; 74:1-380.

7. Bystrom, A; Claesson, R.; Sundqvist, G.: The antibacterial effect of camphorated paramonochlorphenol, camphorated phenol and calcium hydroxide in the treatment of infected root canals. Endod Dent Traumatol. 1985; 1:170.

8. Tronstad, L.; Andreasen, JO; Hasselgren, G.; Kristerson, L.; Riis 1. pH changes in dental tissues following root canal filing with calcium hydroxide. An experimental study in monkeys. J Endod .1981, 7:17-21.

9. Baumgartner, JC; Heggers, JP; Harrison, JW: The incidence of bacteremias

related to endodontic procedures. Non surgical endodontics. J. Endodon 1976; 2:135-40.

10. Debelian GJ, Olsen I, Tronstad L: Bacteremia in conjunction with endodontic therapy. Endodontics & Dental Traumatology. 1995; June; 11: 3: 142-149.

11. Debelian, GJ, Olsen I, Tronstad L: Electrophoresis of whole-cell soluble proteins of microorganisms isolated from bacteremias in endodontic therapy. European Journal of Oral Sciences 1996; October-December;104: 540-546

12. Debelian, GJ, Olsen I, Tronstad L: Anaerobic bacteremia and fungemia in patients undergoing endodontic therapy: an overview. Annals of Periodontology. 1998; 3:281-287.

13. Chaudhry R, Kalra N, Talwar V, Thakur R: Anaerobic flora in endodontic infections The Indian Journal of Medical Research. 1997; 105: 262-265.

14. Baumgartner JC, Falkler WA Jr.: Bacteria in the apical 5 mm of infected root canals. Journal of Endodontics. 1991: 17:380-383.

15. Oguntebi BR: Dentine tubule infection and endodontic therapy implications. International Endodontic Journal. 1994; 27: 218-222.

16. **An excellent book on the dangers of root canals that is scientific and easy to understand:** Kulacz R and Levy T: The Toxic Tooth, Med Fox Pub, 2014, Henderson NV. *Dear Reader*, I highly recommend this book to anyone who has or has been advised to have a root canal. After reading this book, you will have a comprehensive knowledge of how a root canal will seriously affect your health—and it may save your life.

3. <u>Sources of poisoning (electronic poisoning) from aberrant electric currents:</u>

    a. <u>**Disruptive electric currents generated by mixed metals in the mouth:**</u>

Mixed metals in a person's mouth (different metals that were used in a dental restoration—crowns, bridges, etc.) that are in contact with the naturally occurring acid and liquid in the mouth will produce a mini electronic battery that generates a small electric current. The flow of this small electric current somehow is electrically disruptive to the body. I have clinically found that when this situation was corrected by a dentist, the patient reported an immediate and dramatic feeling of improvement while still in the dental chair. This improvement is perceived as a weight lifted from the patient, a clarity—yes, vague and subjective, but tell that to the patient who dramatically and overtly suddenly feels better and immediately and spontaneously comments upon the phenomenon when it occurs.

b. **<u>Electronic poisoning from aberrant surface electronic phenomena</u>:**

See Epilogue 4: "An Electrifying Experience" for a recounting of the most interesting medical experience in my career.

4. **<u>Poisoning from chronic low-level gastrointestinal infections arising out of hypochlorhydria (low stomach acid)</u>.**

A chronic low-level gastrointestinal infection will continuously supply poisons that will disrupt the local gastrointestinal metabolic processes and thus diminish the amount of electrons they supply, thereby lowering the voltage on the absorptive gastrointestinal membrane, and this leads to a "leaky gut."

The following is an explanatory essay on low stomach acid that was excerpted from the book *Zamm AV. Acid reflux, GERD. Amazon Publishing 2021*.

Let's be clear:
The *actual* disease (the *cause* of acid reflux—GERD) was some unknown and mysterious mechanism (unknown and mysterious up to the publication of this book) that prevented the smooth muscle that operates this valve from closing properly. *Stomach acid in the esophagus is not the disease; it is a symptom of the disease—the disease is a muscle problem.*

If you or your doctor are directing your medical activities towards neutralizing this leaked stomach acid by using an anti-antacid or are preventing the stomach from *forming* acid (by using an H_2 histamine-competitive inhibitor or a proton pump inhibitor) you have:

a) not addressed why the valve doesn't close properly;
b) only temporarily made yourself feel better by removing the irritating acid (OK—that's useful but not curative)
c) actually deprived yourself of this valuable and irreplaceable stomach acid (as you shall soon see);

d) have ***actually made yourself worse in the long run*** and

e) you still are left with the disease.

5. <u>Some Premonitory and Depressing Comments about Stomach Acid</u>

The standard "treatment" for GERD, as just mentioned, is a persistent attack on stomach acid.

Is acid really a bad guy? The answer is "yes and no." It's good in the stomach and it's bad in the esophagus. Why is acid good? Cells in the stomach lining (the parietal cells) produce hydrochloric acid. If you don't have enough hydrochloric acid (the technical term is hypochlorhydria), you won't be able to do the following:

1. Digest protein properly, and that results in some degree of malnutrition.
2. Absorb certain essential minerals—more malnutrition.
3. Digest and absorb vitamin B_{12} properly—yet more malnutrition; this is

very serious and common, as elderly people often have insufficient stomach acid. This results in a lower absorption of vitamin B_{12}, and lower bodily vitamin B_{12} results in a decline in one's ability to think clearly because vitamin B_{12} is essential for efficient nerve function. This is one reason why agedness is associated with a decline in clear thinking—and sadly, it is an easily correctible condition that often goes uncorrected (the effective treatment is to prescribe an oral vitamin B_{12} supplement in sufficient strength). I suspect that low vitamin B_{12} will adversely affect the function of macular cells.

4. Defend yourself against invasive bacteria acquired through the normal ingestion of food. Without sufficient stomach acid, these organisms will take up residence in the small intestine, live, multiply, and produce a chronic disease state called "small

intestinal bacterial overgrowth" (SIBO), which leads to:

a. Further interference with digestion, resulting in more poor nutrition.

b. The production and then absorption of bacterial poisons that make the victim chronically feel tired, sick, and "old."

5. Defend yourself against invasive parasites acquired through the normal ingestion of food. This results in the development of multiple chronic parasitic diseases. Organisms that produce such infections can reside in your intestines for life, interfere with digestion, and produce a lifetime of chronically feeling tired, sick, and "old."

6. Avail yourself of the *signaling function* of stomach acid. Normally, when stomach acid along with partially digested food enters your small intestine from the stomach, the acid in

this mixture takes on a second digestive function in the small intestine, a *signaling* function. The acid in this food-acid mixture "tells" the small intestine, the pancreas, and the liver to do their specific jobs in the digestive process.

Think about it: If you are a ACID RELUX-GERD sufferer, do you want to persistently lower the acid in your stomach by taking substances that diminish your stomach acid? Of course not. But if you *stop* your attack on stomach acid, you will have the discomfort and pain of GERD—plus the corrosive effect on your esophagus. If you *continue* your attack on acid, you will have less available stomach acid, and you now know the dangers of that. What to do about this conundrum?

End of Excerpt

Having brought up the subject of low stomach acid (hypochlorhydria) and small

intestine bacterial overgrowth (SIBO), it is appropriate now to suggest some therapy for SIBO:

A. **The Subjective Methods:**
   1. **The use of vitamin C can be ameliorative—but not curative.**
      See Epilogue 5 on vitamin C.
   2. **The use of hot red pepper sauce:**
      Hot red pepper sauce is mildly antimicrobial. The method: use on any food that you find gustatorily pleasing and adjust to taste and use it three times a week and observe how you feel in general; patients tell me that they feel an improved sense of wellbeing and are more energetic. Yes, vague and may not be curative, but still efficacious. This method will have to be used indefinitely.

B. **The Objective Method: This method needs a knowledgeable physician**

Board certified in the specialty of gastroenterology to:

1. Diagnose the presence of SIBO by using the hydrogen breath test.
2. Know which antibiotic to choose to treat SIBO.
3. Recurrences are common.

<u>Giardiasis (an infection with the parasite Giardia lamblia) can disrupt the gastrointestinal membrane's function and lead to food allergy on its own and, additionally, can lead to SIBO</u>.

To diagnose whether a patient has giardiasis:

a. The old method: just looking through a microscope by a trained technician. This method is terrible because it depends on the skill of the examiner. It is not a modern method—I have found this method to be more often misleading than accurate. Dear Reader, if you or your doctor are contemplating a test to determine whether you have giardiasis, **do not use this method.**

b. The modern method: Uses a PCR DNA test. It is an excellent test. This test can be performed as a single test targeting solely Giardia lamblia or this test can be part of a screening test that targets multiple pathogenic microbial targets, which is designated as the.

- Gastrointestinal profile stool multiplex PCR DNA test. For the sake of simplifying things for the reader (as a patient and the attending physician), I will use the information from one company, LabCorp, as a guide for exactly how to order this test:

- Name of test: Gastrointestinal Profile Stool PCR (Multiplex test). The "multiplex" means that this test will test not only for the presence of Giardia lamblia but also for other possible infectious gastrointestinal microorganisms, as since we're doing this test on a patient who has a chronic gastrointestinal inefficiency, you never know what could show up.

- LabCorp test number: LabCorp test number: 183480.
- CPT number: 00970
- LabCorp special instructions: this test needs an Orange "Para pack" collection vial containing Cary-Blair preservative liquid medium. Collection and storage: Room temperature.
- Additional comments:
  1. "PCR" = Polymerase chain reaction
  2. You and your physician will need other instructions, which LabCorp will supply.
  3. There are other laboratory companies that perform this

test. The comments provided here about LabCorp is for the ease of the reader and the attending physician.

c. A comment about therapy for giardiasis: You have two choices:

   i. The inferior method (but unfortunately the common method):

What is currently prescribed: a broad-spectrum antimicrobial medication that is:

   i. Non-specific for Giardia lamblia and not very efficacious (recurrences are common);

   ii. Disruptive to the delicate balance of normal microorganisms in the intestines (the microbiome) by virtue of its broad spectrum.

A comment about metronidazole, a commonly used broad-spectrum medication for this purpose. This medication is available in two forms:

a. The generic form

I have clinically noticed unacceptable undesirable side effects—on one occasion the side effects of generic metronidazole were life-threatening. The problem was related to the inferior manufacturing process of the generic form vis-à-vis the superior quality of the brand form ("Flagyl")—you get what you pay for.

b. The brand form:

The brand name for metronidazole is Flagyl. Patients who had undesirable side effects with generic metronidazole were able to successfully tolerate metronidazole as Flagyl.

I want to make absolutely clear that I have never used metronidazole (generic) or Flagyl (brand) for the treatment of giardiasis. What I used was quinacrine *vida infra*. I only mention all of this as a warning for what you're going to get into for any encounter with physicians who attempt to treat giardiasis with a generic (not brand) broad-spectrum antimicrobial agent.

The use of quinacrine:

- Quinacrine is essentially specific for Giardia lamblia (there are a few other uses, but that doesn't concern us). It has no broad-spectrum antimicrobial activity that would disrupt the delicate gastrointestinal microbiome.
- It has the highest efficacy of all anti-giardia lamblia medications.
- When prescribed as herein delineated, it has been essentially 100% effective.
- The dose I have found to be effective was 100 mg tablets, one with each meal (i.e., 3 times a day) for 21 days (not the lesser number of days that are commonly prescribed, as reoccurrences have been reported with these fewer days of therapy).

- The only contraindication is that some people have a biochemical defect in their enzyme system and cannot tolerate this type of medication, so before initiating a quinacrine program they must be tested by a blood test for the adequate presence of the glucose-6-phosphate dehydrogenase enzyme.
- Watch for the Jarisch-Herxheimer reaction ("Herxheimer" reaction); this can be confused with a side-effect of the medication, which it is not.
- What is the Jarisch-Herxheimer reaction? It's when an antimicrobial medication kills off a large amount of the organism that has been targeted. The cells of the organism are disrupted and the contents of the cells are spilled out into the adjacent environment and are absorbed into the general circulation; these substances are toxic, and they elicit a temporary adverse reaction (the

Jarisch-Herxheimer reaction) until these substances are eliminated from the body. I solve this problem by prescribing a small dose of quinacrine at the beginning of the therapeutic process, specifically ½ tablet once a day for the first two days, then ½ tablet twice a day for the next two days, ½ tablet 3 times a day for the following two days, and then one tablet three times a day thereafter. If the symptoms are too uncomfortable, in addition to the quinacrine also taking two 500 mg. tablets of vitamin C three times a day with food during the Jarisch-Herxheimer reaction will mitigate the symptoms. As soon as the symptoms are gone, vitamin C should be discontinued because vitamin C also has the effect of accelerating the elimination of the quinacrine (and we do need the quinacrine at its maximum therapeutic level).

- **<u>Now here's the bad news:</u>**

Quinacrine was previously sold as the brand name Atabrine by the Winthrop Pharmaceutical Company. When the patent ran out, it was discontinued, and no manufacturer took up the slack. To my way of thinking, this was a disaster, as quinacrine is unique and irreplaceable. But there was a way out of this impediment. There is a type of pharmacist called a compounding pharmacist who will make up medications that are not readily available. A list of these compounding pharmacists can be gotten from either of the two following organizations:

Professional Compounding
Centers of America
Houston TX
1-800-331-2498

Alliance for Pharmaceutical Compounding
Alexandria VA
1-281-933-8400

Hopefully, quinacrine can be obtained in the future—good luck.

6. Xenobiotic poisons: Other entities that decrease metabolic function and thereby result in a decrease in the supply of electrons, thus contributing to an induction of food allergy:

   a. **Inhalants: Xenobiotic inhalants** Chemicals such as petroleum-derived substances, automobile effluent, chemicals commonly found in the home such as floor wax, chemicals used in the clothes dryer, the gas stove effluent.

   b. **Ingestants: Xenobiotic Ingestants:** Chemicals found in foods: insecticide residues, preservatives, food colorings, chlorine added to communal drinking water.

     Hint: You can remove these agricultural poisons from foods by washing these fruits and vegetables ***with a detergent*** (*vide supra*).

7. Genetic causes of lower voltage:

Some individuals are born with a defective secretory IgA molecule (see Epilogues 2 and 3)

Epilogues

Epilogue 1

SELENIUM, OBSERVATIONS AND REFERENCES

In my medical practice I advised patients to take *inorganic* selenium in the form of sodium selenite solution (the only source of inorganic selenium that I have been able to find is the Allergy Research Group company). Only the *inorganic* form of selenium and not the organic form has the ability to substantially bind and chemically inactivate mercury. The term "organic" is a technical term in the academic subject of chemistry and relates to selenium being part of a **carbon-containing** molecule, and this is not to be confused with "organic" as in organic farming. The organic (carbon-containing) form of selenium is widely sold and is **less effective** than the inorganic form.

In this ***inorganic*** form selenium has the ability to similarly bind and chemically inactivate other metallic poisons such as cadmium, arsenic, and some other heavy metals that are unavoidably encountered in our environment.

Selenium is an essential nutrient. My patients have found that selenium in this form was salubrious when used as herein described (vide infra).

THE FOLLOWING IS AN INSTRUCTIONAL FORM THAT I HAVE PROVIDED TO PATIENTS IN CONJUNCTION WITH MY PRESCRIBING SELENIUM

<u>HOW AND WHY TO USE SELENIUM</u>

Some chemically sensitive and mercury-poisoned patients improve with the use of selenium. The response to the use of selenium can be divided into three clinical groups.

<u>GROUP 1</u>: They experience immediate benefit within the first few days. These patients

feel better, stronger, and are more tolerant of xenobiotic chemicals.

<u>GROUP 2</u>: They improve slowly. These patients may not be aware of their slow progress until they realize that they can tolerate tobacco smoke and other xenobiotic exposures without deleterious results. Their symptoms decrease gradually in duration and magnitude.

<u>GROUP 3</u>: They initially react in an apparently *unfavorable* way. These patients are generally the most sensitive, the most debilitated, and those most in need of selenium but they are initially unable to deal with it. It takes longer for these patients to receive benefit. It often can take these ultrasensitive patients up to six months of being free of their mercury fillings before they start to tolerate and benefit from selenium. At that point they find that they can begin to increase the amount of selenium they are taking. This may be because selenium

combines with heavy metals, forming compounds that. these sensitive patients may not tolerate.

Selenium is not a medicine. It is not a prescription item. It is an <u>essential nutrient</u> and is sold over the-counter. It is found in many over-the-counter vitamin preparations. The difference between taking selenium in a chemically pure liquid form and merely taking a selenium tablet. or selenium mixed with other vitamins and minerals is that by taking selenium in solution, considerably more selenium is absorbed.

Selenium is needed in very small amounts. This means that other minerals, which are found in relatively huge quantities when compared with the amount of selenium present, "overwhelm" the absorption of the small amount of selenium, and the patient who takes selenium in a tablet form or in a vitamin-mineral mixture or with food is able to obtain very little of the selenium he swallowed.

Selenium must be taken on an <u>empty stomach</u>. Other substances found in foods bind to selenium and prevent its absorption.

<u>Selenium is essential for everyone, but it is especially important to patients who have difficulty dealing with environmental xenobiotics and are mercury-poisoned from dental fillings.</u>

   I. <u>Selenium binds with and neutralizes poisonous heavy metals</u> found in the environment such as mercury, arsenic, and cadmium; this is especially helpful in regard to the mercury that leaches out of dental fillings.

   2. <u>Selenium is an essential part of the xenobiotic (harmful chemical) detoxification system:</u>

      (a) Selenium is part of glutathione peroxidase, an important enzyme that the body uses to detoxify harmful chemicals.

      (b) Mercury leaching out from

dental fillings produces another problem in addition to supplying mercury as a poison. Mercury binds with selenium, <u>thus depriving the patient of available selenium</u>. The patient becomes "selenium starved" and can no longer manufacture adequate amounts of glutathione peroxidase. Supplying selenium overcomes this problem.

HOW TO TAKE SELENIUM SOLUTION

<u>REMEMBER: ALWAYS TAKE SELENIUM SOLUTION ON AN EMPTY STOMACH! !</u>

Transfer some selenium solution from the stock bottle you purchased at the pharmacy into the glass dropper bottle using a <u>plastic</u> funnel. Do not use a metal funnel, as it may react with the selenium.

For GROUPS 1 and 2: When you get up in the morning:

1. Dissolve the drop(s) (see below) in 2 oz. water
2. Drink the selenium solution before you swallow any food or take any vitamins or medication
3. By the time you are ready to have your breakfast (after 5-10 minutes later) you will have absorbed a good deal of the selenium, without the interference or neutralization by any stomach contents.

Suggested schedule for Groups 1 and 2 to take selenium

Before Breakfast		**Before Breakfast**	
Day 1	1 drop	Day 8	15 drops
Day 2	2 drops	Day 9	17 drops
Day 3	4 drops	Day 10	20 drops
Day 4	7 drops	Day 11 and thereafter	
Day 5	9 drops	Take 1/2 dropperful	
Day 6	11 drops	+ 1/2 dropperful	
Day 7	13 drops	+ 1/2 dropperful	

(A total of 1 1/2 droppers. Using 3 half droppersful is more practical than trying to fill a dropper completely, as the air trapped in the glass tube in the dropper may prevent complete filling.) <u>On Day 11 and each morning thereafter</u>: Continue at this dose—you will have reached the daily maintenance dose.

For GROUP 3: The patients in Group 3 (the most sensitive patients), should increase the dose very slowly; it may take weeks to months to substantially increase the daily dose, and they may never achieve a full dose.

Addendum

Even on small doses of selenium, some patients with arthritis become symptom-free (Veterinarians have used selenium to treat arthritis in dogs for years.).

Selenium is protective against cancer. Some references:

Willett WC et al. Prediagnostic serum selenium and risk of cancer. Lancet II: 130-4, July 16, 1983.

Shamberger RJ and Willis CE. Selenium Distribution and Human Cancer Mortality, Critical Reviews in Laboratory Sciences 2:211-21 (June 1971).

Shamberger R. Relationship of Selenium to Cancer: Inhibiting Effect of Selenium on Carcinogenesis, Journal of the National Cancer Institute 44:931-36 (April 1970)

Some comments and peer-reviewed references documenting that other scientists feel the same way about selenium:

1. Selenium is involved with the enzymes of thyroid metabolism, glutathione metabolism, and other multiple ancillary enzyme systems.

2. A unique and comprehensive review article on selenium is: Fairweather-Tate SJ et al: Selenium in human health and disease in Antioxidants and Redox Signaling Vol 14 No. 7, 2011 (Mary Ann Liebert, Inc., publishers). Reader, please note that, in addition to this fine comprehensive review article, its bibliography is a treasure trove of excellent references.

3. Combs JR, GF et al. An analysis of cancer prevention by selenium (Review) *Biofactors* 2001;14(1-4):153-9. PMID: 11568452.

4. Schrauzer GN. Selenium and cancer: A review *Bioinorg Chem. 1976;5(3):275-81. PMID: 769840.*

5. Ganther HE. Selenium metabolism selenoproteins and mechanisms of cancer prevention: Complexities with thioredoxin reductase (Review). *Carcinogenesis* 1999 Sep;20(9):1657-66. PMID 10469608.

6. Schrauzer GN. Selenium. Mechanistic aspects of anticarcinogenic action (Review). *Biol Trace Elem Res*. Apr-Jun 1992;33:51-62. PMID 1379460.

7. Schrauzer GN. Selenium and selenium-antagonistic elements in nutritional cancer prevention (Review). *Crit Rev Biotechnol*. 2009;29(1):10-7. PMID 19514899.

8. Schrauzer GN. Effects of selenium antagonists on cancer susceptibility: New aspects of chronic heavy metal toxicity (Review). *J UOEH*. 1987;Mar 20;9 Suppl:208-15. PMID 3299603.

9. Jukes, TH: When Friends or Patients Ask About... Mercury in Fish. JAMA. 1975;233:1001-1002.

10. Parizek J, Ostadalova, I: The protective effective effects of small amounts of selenite in sublimate intoxication. Experientia .1967; 23:142-3.

11. Ganther HE, Goudie C, Sunde ML, et al: Selenium: Relation to decreased

toxicity of methyl-mercury added to diets containing tuna. Science. 1972; 175:1122-1124.

12. Koeman JH, Peeters WHM, Koudstaal-Hol CHM, et al: Mercury-selenium correlations in marine mammals. Nature. 1973; 245:385-386.

13. Kosta L, Byrne AR, Zelenko V: Correlation between selenium and mercury in man following exposure to inorganic mercury. Nature. 1975; 4:238-239.

Epilogue 2

ELECTRONICS, THE LEAKY GUT, AND FOOD ALLERGY—WHAT'S THE CONNECTION— AN ABBREVIATED VERSION

The following article, Zamm AV: Letter: Is food allergy a failure of secretory IgA, a gatekeeper that is an electronic transistor? *J Ortho Med*. Vol 29, No 2, 201486-87 (reprinted by permission), will serve as a tutorial for Epilogue 3.

A myriad of molecules is presented to the absorptive surface of the gastrointestinal tract; this surface either absorbs or blocks absorption of molecules by a gatekeeping mechanism that has never been explained.

(A) The Gatekeeper

"All of science is either physics or stamp collecting"—Ernest Rutherford (1851-1937) Nobel Prize Laureate.

It is conjectured that: (1) the gatekeeper

is an electronic transistor in the form of a secretory IgA molecule that is assembled on
site in the gastrointestinal lining; (2) the secretory piece, typical of transistors' familiar
structure, operates together with exogenous
energy to constrain electrons to flow in one
direction; (3) because this molecule is a "sand-
wich" composed of two serum IgA molecules
connected by a single central secretory IgA
piece, it can be polarized to hold an electrical
charge at each end of the molecule.[1]

For the reader's ease in orienting to the
electronic concepts referred to in this cor-
respondence, I refer the reader to my article[1,] (PubMed PMID number 24068871).
This article painlessly imparts the essential
information necessary in understanding the
electronics involved, and is a recounting of
the scientific odyssey that led to making
the counterintuitive connection between
the seemingly unconnected entities of solar
wind, electronics, secretory IgA, and food
allergy. I believe the reader will enjoy the
voyage in the article and find it interesting

and useful in explaining the details of how the gastrointestinal tract works by acting as an electronic device.

(B) The Gastrointestinal Sorting Process

It is proposed that: (1) these polarized electronic transistor molecules congregate into a reticulum that results in the formation of an electronic sieve. The size of the electronic apertures in this sieve determines, by size, the resultant passage or blockage of passage of molecules (food and other particles); (2) The electronic size of the apertures is a function of energy from the solar wind impinging upon the secretory piece. The solar energy falling on the secretory piece modulates its one-way-electron-passage property, in a manner characteristic of transistors and thus controls the magnitude of the electrical charge that accumulates at each end of the secretory IgA molecule; (3) The more solar energy falling on the secretory piece, the greater will be the "one-way" character of the secretory piece, the greater will be the charge accumulated at the ends of the molecule, the smaller will be the electronic aperture and, hence, the smaller the size of the molecules that will be permitted to pass through the aperture; (4) The degree of efficacy of the gatekeeper in capturing energy from the solar wind and, as a result, storing an electrical charge at each end of the secretory IgA molecule is a function of the intrinsic genetically determined electronic efficiency of a secretory IgA molecule vs. the impact of a disease that disrupts the electronic function of this molecule.[1]

(C) The Clinical Consequences when the Gatekeeper Electronically Fails

1. *Allergies:* If food allergens are inappropriately allowed to pass the gatekeeper into the bloodstream, the result can be the development of food allergies. Clinical manifestations of food allergies (other than the conventional obvious ones of skin

rashes, rhinitis, sinusitis, asthma, diarrhea, etc.) can be:

a. Myocardial infarction[2]
b. Vascular phenomena[3,4]
c. Neurological phenomena: migraines, epilepsy, depression, attention deficit hyperactivity disorder[5]
d. Multisystemal phenomena[6]

2. *Depressed immune system:* Absorption of food allergens produces a drop in the white cell count.[7] A depressed white cell count renders the individual less able to defend itself against foreign invaders such as microorganisms or cancer cells.

If these diseases are re-examined and viewed as electronic dysfunction, then prevention and treatment could involve the use of salubrious electronic modalities that enhance the electronics of the electronic sieve process—an option not entertained in the current practice of medicine.

References

1. Zamm AV: A clinical case-based hypothesis: Secretory IgA operates as an electronic transistor controlling the selection or rejection of molecules in the absorption process in the lumen of the gastrointestinal tract. *Clin Exp Gastroenterol,* 2013; 6:177-184.
2. Davies DF, Elwood PC: Letter: Food antibodies and myocardial infarction. *Lancet,* 1974; 2:219-229.
3. Rea W: Environmentally triggered small vessel vasculitis. *Annals of Allergy,* 1977;38:245-251.
4. Glynn LE: Vascular allergy and its systemic manifestations. *Proc R Soc Med,* 1964;57:399.
5. Speer F: *Allergy of the Nervous System.* Springfield IL. Charles C. Thomas Publisher. 1970.
6. Brostoff J, Challacombe SJ: *Food Allergy and Intolerance.* Eastbourne, UK. Bailliere Tindall. 1987.

7. Cohen SG: Firsts in Allergy: IV. The contributions of Arthur F. Coca, M.D. (1875-1959). (1875-1959). *N Engl Reg Allergy Proc,* 1985;6:285-293.

8. Vaughan WT, Food allergens III. The leukopenic index, preliminary report, *J Allergy*, 5:601, 1934.

Epilogue 3

ELECTRONICS, THE LEAKY GUT, AND FOOD ALLERGY—WHAT'S THE CONNECTION?—AN EXPANDED VERSION

The following introductory remarks will serve to explain the herein-cited article (PMID number 24068871) that is essential reading on this subject:

Food allergy results from an electronic failure that produces a leaky gut (a failure of an electronic sieve that's supposed to function as a selective filtration device). This failure results from a defective electronic gatekeeper (more specifically, a failure of the secretory IgA molecule, which functions as an electronic transistor, the actual gatekeeper.

Dear Interior Designer: there is a peculiar glitch in the program we are using so that in the preceding paragraph the small letters 1. Zamm AV: A clinical case-based

hypothesis.... Exist. We cannot figure out what they're doing there, how to isolate them, or how to remove them. I hope you can delete them. With great thanks.

Multiple such molecules in aggregate form this electronic sieve.
Food allergy exists because this electronic sieve has lost some of its electronic ability to correctly select which molecules to absorb **into** the bloodstream from the digested food in the gastrointestinal tract and which molecules to **keep out** of the bloodstream from the food in the gastrointestinal tract. It now allows some "wrong" (too large) molecules to enter the bloodstream, and these "wrong" molecules instigate an allergic response because they are too large, and under these circumstances the body views all such large molecules as being foreign invaders. For more (and startling) information, read the following recommended article (it can be a fun read and will answer many questions,

some of which you may not yet have even formulated).

Yes, it's a long title, but your journey in reading this article will not only be fun but reveal amazing facts that I have not yet told you—trust me on this.

Zamm A: A Clinical Case-Based Hypothesis. Secretory IgA Operates as an Electronic Transistor Controlling the Selection or Rejection of Molecules in the Absorption Process in the Lumen of the Gastrointestinal Tract. *Clin Exp Gastroenterol*. 201 6:177-184. DOI: 10.2147/CEG.S47772. PMID: 24068871.

This article is in PubMed, a free data-base that is run by the U.S. Government; it is composed of peer-reviewed scientific professional medical articles.

This entire article can be accessed from PubMed at no expense. Here's how you do it:

1. Use your computer and go on Google
2. When on Google, search for "Google Scholar Advanced Search"

3. When on "Google Scholar Advanced Search," search for: "PubMed 24068871;" it's quite simple and sounds worse than it is.

The entire article will miraculously appear for free, and you will have what you need to answer your questions—even questions that you have not yet imagined.

Tip: If you like, you can skip reading the technical section called Methods and Materials. But for the rest of the article, I have confidence in you (after all, you have come this far with me on our journey)—it will be a fun read.

Epilogue 4

AN ELECTRIFYING EXPERIENCE

As you have figured out by now, I am fascinated by the relationship between electronics and biochemistry. The following case report is about this relationship and is the most interesting case of my 60 years of practice as a medical specialist.

An electrifying experience: Chart #38510
RALPH, a 39-year-old obese man, visited me professionally because of an itching, widespread, and red scaling skin condition. Five years prior to this visit, at the same time that this skin condition appeared, he developed an unexplained increase in his weight of 100 pounds, elevated blood pressure, muscle and joint pains, sleep disturbance, nasal congestion, diabetes, and other mysterious symptoms.

An extensive history, a complete physical examination, and a variety of laboratory tests revealed only one odd clue: Five years ago, just prior to the onset of his medical deterioration, Ralph began wearing a metal "M.I.A" ("Missing in Action") bracelet on his right wrist. Some people wear these bracelets to honor soldiers who were M.I.A. in the Vietnam War. During these five years, Ralph never took off that bracelet. I told Ralph that before we initiate an even more complex investigation, we should direct our attention to the only clue we had—the five-year history of contact of his skin with metal. I asked him to remove the bracelet and to keep it off until his next scheduled office visit, one month hence.

When I saw him one month later, this was his report: "Two days after I removed the bracelet, the itching stopped for the first time in five years and after two weeks, the rash was almost gone." At this one-month post-bracelet-removal period, I verified that his rash was indeed gone, except for a few barely visible pinkish areas. In addition, he was "spontaneously" losing some of his excessive weight, and many of his five-year-old maladies had improved or had disappeared.

To my way of thinking, we had a **crime** (a previously healthy man who suddenly develops an unexplained five-year episode of deteriorating health) and we had a **criminal** (the metal bracelet).

How did the criminal commit this crime?

On the face of it, this story is hard to comprehend, yet when you think about it, we are all intuitively aware that we are affected by electrical phenomena—even if we don't call it electrical. We feel more energetic when we are surrounded by more small *negative* atmospheric air ions than small *positive* atmospheric air ions. **(Air ions are electrically charged particles in the air.)**

1. There are more negative than positive atmospheric air ions with *sea* breezes, the spray from fountains, mountainous areas on sunny days

and when it starts to rain. On the other hand, we feel no benefit at the beach when a sea breeze switches to a *land* breeze or on cloudy days—both conditions in which there is no surplus of negative atmospheric air ions.

2. Some people can tell when a storm is approaching: they experience joint pains, fatigue, and even headache *before* the storm arrives (more *positive* than negative atmospheric air ions) and experience exhilaration and relief when the rain starts (the reverse occurs: more *negative* than positive atmospheric air ions).

   Machines that produce negative ions are deceptively sold in a futile attempt to duplicate the beneficial effect of an elevated level of negative ions when found in nature. Unfortunately, many of these machines are not only useless but additionally produce ozone, a toxic gas.

3. Some people are very sensitive to various subtle forms of electrical phenomena. Minor electrical disturbances, such as metal in contact with their skin, seems to short-circuit some kind of electrical pathway and produce strange results—maybe it's a kind of "wrong acupuncture."

Some people wear copper bracelets and they report that they perceive less pain from their arthritis. (They do *feel* better but *aren't* really better—their illness continues.)

The Nobel LaureateAlbert Szent-Györgyi in his book "Bioelectronics" said, "the living cell is essentially an electrical device" (and, hence, I say is subject to being affected by ambient electrical exposure).

Electrical phenomena and their effect on living things is a controversial subject. There is much discussion as to whether other electrical phenomena affect us, such as high voltage electrical transmission wires, various types of radio waves, and cell phones.

I often wonder if metal placed in the skin—such as earrings or metal skin piercings (the latest fashion) affects some individuals. It would make an interesting scientific study.

Apparently, in removing the metal bracelet, Ralph removed some electrical disturbance. I leave it to university-based scientists to provide a scientific explanation of the physics of what happened.

In order to understand what happens in the world that we personally experience on a day-to-day basis, we must recognize that these observed events are merely consequences of a basic, often mysterious hidden world of physics.

I believe that Professor Ernest Rutherford, Nobel Prize Laureate (1851-1937), in his iconoclastic and epigrammic quip, summed it up when he said, "all science is either physics or stamp collecting."

I believe that Professor Szent-Györgyi is implying that many of the medical problems patients suffer—such as the *symptoms* of pain, fatigue, depression, and painful joints and *diseases* such as infection, cancer, and heart ailments—can be viewed as end products of electrical phenomena and that therapeutic solutions to these problems may one day be electronic solutions.

Some thoughts about the body and electrical conductivity that I think about vis-à-vis my experience with this patient:

A. <u>Tattoos:</u>

Tattoos involve the introduction into the skin of potentially electrically conductive materials.

Question One: Does this distort the electrical conductivity of the recipient's skin?

Question Two: How would an electrically sensitive person (like Ralph) be affected by a tattoo?

B. <u>Jewelry:</u>

Metallic jewelry involves the application of metal to the skin surface or insertion of metal into the skin (earrings, piercings)

Question One: *vide supra*—ditto?

Question Two: *vide supra*—ditto?

C. <u>Dental Restorations:</u>

Some dental restorations involve the use of metals:

Question One: *vide supra*—ditto?

Question Two: Vide supra—ditto?

Dear Reader, Now is the time to remember the previous discussion of dental "mixed metals" that appeared in the interior of this book.

I suggest to my patients to have their dentist select non-electrically conductive restorative materials such as plastic polymers, porcelain, or the very strong and durable zirconium dioxide.

D. <u>Here's an idea for a PhD candidate to do a research paper or a college professor to get the Nobel Prize—or at least do some good:</u>

1. Find a group of electrically sensitive individuals (by clinical history)

2. Analyze their secretory IgA molecule. Dear Reader, see a discussion
   of the secretory IgA molecule in the
   PUBMED Article No. 24068871 (*vide
   supra)* for an explanation of the secretory IgA molecule).

   The scientist should analyze the
physical structure and electronic
function of the secretory IgA molecule in an electrically sensitive person and compare it to the secretory
IgA molecule in a non-electrically
sensitive person.

My bet: the secretory IgA molecules
from each of these two types of individuals (electrically and non-electrically sensitive) will somehow be
different.

The individual with the electrical sensitivity and the abnormal
secretory IgA molecule will have
food allergies—among other health

issues (see "Common Complaints," Appendix I)_

Not only do these ideas engender new avenues of approach for dealing with illness, but also engender possibilities for commercial exploitation of these ideas that might benefit a variety of sufferers from various health issues—just some ideas that float around in my head.

E: <u>Where would a potential scientist-researcher find such a cohort of electrically sensitive individuals (EMF, electromagnetic field-sensitive individuals) to do this research?</u>

Here's how I would do it: I would contact a commercial enterprise that sells EMF-protective devices to electrically sensitive individuals, discuss this project with them, and see if they would contact their customers to volunteer to participate.

There is such a well-established company:
"The Less EMF Company"
776B Watervliet Shaker Road
Latham NY 12110
USA

Contact Information:
Telephone: (Toll-free USA): 1-888-537-7363
Telephone (Outside the USA):
+1 (518) 608-6479
Fax: 1 (309) 422-4355
Email: **lessemf@lessemf.com**
website: www.lessemf.com

F. <u>It's Not a New Idea:</u>

The application of an electroconductive material to the skin, as in the use of metal needles or electrostimulation in acupuncture. has been known for years to be able to induce profound changes in subjects; the exact etiological explanation of how this works has never been entirely explained.

Every time an electrically conductive substance is introduced on or within the body, the provider and the recipient (the victim) should recite out loud and in unison the philosopher/epigrammist Voltaire's (1691-1778) prescient words of guidance: *"physicians take medicines of which they know little and put* them into patients of which they know less...."

Epilogue 5

THREE WEIRD FOOD ALLERGIES TO MAMMALIAN MEAT— NATURE'S PRACTICAL JOKES

1. Pork: The Pork-Cat Allergy Syndrome: Through an accident of nature, there is some similarity between the structure of a molecule found in cats and the structure of a molecule found in pigs. A person who is allergic to cats can also be allergic to pig (pork). If you live with a cat or did so in the past, you could be allergic to pork and yet not know it and have resultant mysterious symptoms (see "Common Complaints" in the Appendix for a list of possible symptoms).

Who would ever connect a friendly housecat with the possibility of an allergy to food? It's a weird world.

Here's a summary-mnemonic of a projected possibility:

Cat → allergy to cat →unexpected symptoms and location

2. Tick bites producing allergy to mammalian meat: pork, beef, and lamb:

   a. The sensitization process:

The bite of certain ticks (the Lone Star Tick in the USA and the "paralysis tick" in Australia) injects a peculiar molecule (the alpha-gal molecule) into the recipient. The human recipient immunologically views this molecule as a dangerous foreign invader and reacts allergically and defensively against it. This process is called sensitization. This molecule is not found in humans but is found in some mammals: pig (pork), cow (beef), and sheep (lamb).

   b. The reactive process:

Here's what happens now that the human has been sensitized to the alpha-gal molecule by developing antibodies against it:

When, after being sensitized by the bite, the sensitized human again immunologically encounters this alpha-gal molecule—this time by eating the meat of these mammals—the human recognizes this molecule from the past and again views it as a foreign invader, i.e. views the alpha-gal molecule as if it were as an invasion of a dangerous microbe, which it is not. The human now allergically reacts to the alpha-gal molecule within the pork, beef, or lamb that was eaten and doesn't cognitively connect this reaction to the original sensitization, the bite. Now the sensitized human should avoid eating these meats but doesn't know to do so.

In summary, it is possible for the bite of a tick to instigate food allergy and, hence, a multiplicity of symptoms and locations if the person continues to eat these meats.

A thought that comes to mind: Could it be possible that the poor sufferers of so-called "chronic Lyme disease" have some connection with this alpha-gal problem and are actually suffering from a food allergy—just a thought.

3. Another idiosyncratic adventure into food allergy: Pork, beef, and lamb

Here's another nuisance that can plague us: A peculiar molecule found in most mammals (but **not** found in humans) is the Neu5Ge molecule. When a person eats pork, beef, or lamb and is exposed to this Neu5Ge molecule, a similar process of "sensitization and reaction" that was described in Number 2 (above) can occur with the exposure to this molecule by eating these meats.

Epilogue 6

SOME SURPRISING OBSERVATIONS ON FOOD ALLERGY AND IDEAS FOR RESEARCH

1. **Glaucoma: the removal of food allergens from allergic patients' diets has been reported to normalize intraocular pressure in patients having glaucoma:**
   Berens C, Gerard L, Cumming E. Allergy in glaucoma. Chapter XXVII in Coca AF. *Familial Nonreaginic food allergy. Lyle Stuart Secaucus NJ 4th ed. 1982.*

2. **Infections and cancer: Food allergy lowers the white blood cell count.**
   This phenomenon that food allergy can lower the number of white blood cells in the blood was first noted in: Vaughan WT, Food allergens III. The leukopenic index, preliminary report, *J Allergy*, 5:601, 1934.

A lowered white count is a comorbid finding that predisposes to lowered defense by the immune system against invading bacteria and cancer.

Reminder: see a similar discussion on the lowering of T-cells (white blood cells) by mercury poisoning in the Eggleston reference (*vide supra*).

Yes, what I'm saying is that food allergy by suppressing the blood white cell count can be a predisposing factor for a poor ability to deal with infection or cancer.

Appendices

Appendix 1

COMMON COMPLAINTS THAT THE SUFFERER MAY NOT ATTRIBUTE TO A HYPERSENSITIVITY TO FOODS AND/OR INHALANTS

NERVE AND MUSCLE PROBLEMS

1. Fainting
2. Blurred vision
3. Unexplained hyperactivity
4. Headache
5. Dizziness

MOOD CHANGES

1. Unexplained anxiety
2. Unwarranted excitability
3. Unexplained irritability
4. Hostility
5. Aggression
6. Insomnia
7. Restlessness
8. Difficulty concentrating
9. Difficulty thinking
10. Mental confusion

11. Grogginess
12. Decreased reading comprehension
13. Forgetfulness
14. Difficulty recalling words
15. Depression
16. Loss of interest in work or former activities or hobbies
17. Crying spells
18. Tendency for fixed ideas; recycling or repeating of ideas
19. Antisocial behavior
20. Thoughts of suicide

ORGAN AND SYSTEMS PROBLEMS

1. Skin
   Rashes
   Excessive perspiration
2. Eyes
   Burning
   Itching
   Excessive tearing
   Feeling of heaviness and pressure within eyes
3. Ears
   Dizziness (Meniere's syndrome)
   Decreased hearing
   Buzzing in ears (tinnitus)

"Plugged"
ears (swollen
eustachian
tubes)

4. Nose
Nasal
obstruction
Sinus
congestion
Sneezing
(Rubbing nose
upward is a sign
of allergy)

5. Throat
Hoarseness
"Itching"
throat (leading
to clucking
sounds)
Sore throat
Excessive mucus

6. Lungs
Wheezing
Coughing

7. Cardiovascular
Palpitations
Flushing

8. Gastrointestinal
Nausea
Loss of appetite
Voracious
appetite
Weight gain
Chronic obesity
Excessive thirst

9. Genitourinary
Urgent
urination
Frequent
urination
Bedwetting
Vaginal itching
Excessively
painful
menstruation

10. Muscular-skeletal
Joint pains
Uncertain gait

GENERAL PHYSICAL PROBLEMS

1. Fatigue (physical or mental)
2. Loss of former energy ("getting old")
3. Weakness
4. Edema (swelling)
5. Pallor
6. Inappropriate chilliness or excessive warmth
7. Excessive perspiration without fever

© 1989 Alfred Zamm, M.D.

HOW TO DEAL WITH YOUR FOOD ALLERGY

Now that a diagnosis of food allergy has been made, what does this mean in terms of your daily living habits? Will you have to stop eating this food? This instructional section will clarify your situation now and will be a source of information and a guide in your future care.

I. The Effect of Family Relationship

The food to which you have been found to be allergic belongs to a taxonomic family; that is, it is closely related to other, similar foods. The best-known example, the "orange family" has in it grapefruit, lemon, lime, tangerine, and a number of other, similar foods (see Appendix III). Hence, to those patients who are allergic to the whole family (in this example, the orange family), any one of these foods will produce a problem. In this case, orange or lemon or grapefruit, etc., will all be troublesome, and the entire family should be avoided.

On the other hand, not everyone is allergic to an entire family. Many individuals have an allergy only to that specific food. In this second example, a person could be allergic to only orange and not to grapefruit or lemon, etc., Hence, some patients can eat a single member of a family, while others can eat only some members of a family. You may ask, to which group do I belong? The only way to know is to try each member of the family one week apart and see whether symptoms develop.

II. The Effect of Form

The food to which you have been found to be allergic may be utilizable in one or two forms: uncooked and/or cooked. You may have customarily eaten a food uncooked or cooked all your life and, hence, by repetitive exposure, became allergic to that form only and not to the other. Hence, knowledge of your previous lifestyle may allow you to utilize this form of food in the other, unaccustomed form, without producing allergic symptoms. For example, you may have been found to be allergic to orange. Your mode of living may have included the use of orange as a fresh fruit or a frozen juice. Cooked orange may never have appeared in your diet; hence, you may never have developed an allergy to the cooked form. To test this, you should try the cooked form. The canning process utilizes heat; therefore, the juice has been "cooked."

III. The Effect of Concomitance

You may find that you can tolerate the food to which you have been found to be allergic by itself, but not in combination with exposure to other allergens (either another food or another inhalant). For example, you may be allergic orange only when together with wheat. But either food alone may or may not produce allergic symptoms. When allergic symptoms are produced by two things together and not by either one taken separately, this state is called concomitance.

Concomitant reactions can also occur when a food and a non-food are simultaneously part of an exposure. An example of this would be when both a food and an inhalant (pollen, house dust, mold, etc.) are part of the exposure together. Since inhalants occur in seasonal patterns, in certain cases a patient may tolerate a food in one season and not another. An example would be a patient who can consume orange in all seasons except the ragweed season. In summary, you should test a food and observe if you can tolerate it during all seasons.

The following is a very brief, rough description of allergy seasons in the Northeastern United States; other regions will vary.

Spring:	March to May	Tree pollens
Summer:	Last week in May to last week in July	Grass pollens
Fall:	Mid-August to Mid-September	Ragweed pollens
Spring to frost/snow:	Spring to early winter	Mold
Winter to Spring:	Mid-September (heating season starts) (Heating season ends)	House dust

Remember: concomitance can be a <u>food plus a food</u> or a <u>food plus an inhalant.</u>

IV. The Effect of Dosage in Time and Space:

A. <u>The Effect of Dosage in Time:</u>

Fixed or cyclical allergic response: You may find that you are able to tolerate a food "once in a while" but not every day. This means that you are experiencing a cyclical type of response; that is, your sensitivity is highest after an exposure and lowest after some time has elapsed (*i.e.,* a "rest). By giving your body a "rest" between exposures, you can take advantage of this situation and consume the food in an intermittent pattern. By experience, you will be able to determine how often you can consume this food (for example, every other day, once a week, once a month, etc.).

On the other hand, some individuals have a fixed type of allergic response. These individuals react in a similar manner, even if they have given their body a rest. That is, they *always* react unfavorably and hence, can never consume the food they are allergic to, no matter how long the rest period.

Of course, each person is different, and hence you will have to determine what your situation is.

B. The Effect of Space:

Not only is the planning of your food exposures—by having rest periods in between—important, but the *amount* (that is, the *volume*) of food taken at each exposure also can be a critical factor. For example, the consumption of the equivalent of one orange a day may be tolerable and not produce symptoms. More than one orange a day, however, may produce symptoms. The way to tell is by trial and error.

V. The Effect of Substitution

Often the taste—and perhaps the nutritional quality—of a substitute (a familiarly unrelated food) will satisfy the dietary and gustatory requirements of the food-allergic patient. Example: in the case of an orange-sensitive patient, pomegranate juice or pineapple juice and the addition of vitamin C tablets may satisfy the taste and nutritional needs without great inconvenience.

In summary, by recognizing the influence of the factors of 1) family relationship 2) form (cooked vs raw) 3) concomitance (effect of other foods or seasons) 4) time and space (frequency or amount of use) and 5) substitution on your allergic state, you will be able to circumvent some of the problems of food allergy.

©1996 Alfred V. Zamm, M.D.

Appendix 3

DIETARY TAXONOMY

1. **Mushrooms**
2. **Grass Family**
   a. bamboo
   b. barley
   c. wheat
   d. rye
   e. oats
   f. rice
   g. millet
   h. sugar cane
   i. sorghum
3. **Chinese Water Chestnuts**
4. **Palm Family**
   a. coconut
   b. sago
   c. date
5. **Taro, Poi**
6. **Pineapple**
7. **Garlic Family**
   a. garlic
   b. onion
   c. leek
   d. chives
   e. asparagus
8. **Sarsaparilla**
9. **Banana**
10. **Ginger Family**
    a. ginger
    b. turmeric
11. **Arrowroot**
12. **Vanilla**
13. **Black pepper**
14. **Walnut Family**
    a. walnut
    b. pecan
    c. hickory
15. **Beechnut Family**
    a. beechnut

b. chestnut

16. **Mulberry Family**
    a. mulberry
    b. fig
    c. breadfruit

17. **Macadamia nut**

18. **Buckwheat Family**
    a. buckwheat
    b. rhubarb

19. **Spinach Family**
    a. spinach
    b. Swiss chard
    c. common beet
    d. sugar beet

20. **Pawpaw**

21. **Nutmeg Family**
    a. nutmeg
    b. mace

22. **Avocado Family**
    a. avocado
    b. cinnamon
    c. sassafras

23. **Cabbage Family**
    a. cabbage
    b. Brussels sprouts
    c. broccoli
    d. cauliflower
    e. kale
    f. collards
    g. kohlrabi
    h. mustard*
    i. turnip
    j. rutabaga

24. **Strawberry Family**
    a. strawberry
    b. raspberry
    c. blackberry

25. **Apple Family**
    a. apple
    b. pear

26. **Plum Family**
    a. plum (incl. prune)
    b. peach

c. apricot

d. almond

e. cherry

27. <u>Gooseberry Family</u>

a. gooseberry

b. currant

28. <u>Gum acacia</u>

29. <u>Peanut Family</u>

a. peanut

b. pea*

c. beans*

d. lentils

e. licorice

f. gum tragacanth

30. <u>Citrus Family</u>

a. orange

b. grapefruit

c. lemon

d. lime

e. tangerine

f. citron

g. kumquat

31. <u>Tapioca</u>

32. <u>Litchi nut</u>

33. <u>Cashew Family</u>

a. cashew

b. pistachio

c. mango

34. <u>Maple Sugar</u>

35. <u>Grapes*</u>

36. <u>Okra Family</u>

a. okra

b. cottonseed

37. <u>Chocolate Family</u>

a. chocolate

b. cola

c. gum karaya

38. <u>Tea</u>

39. <u>Papaya</u>

40. <u>Guava Family</u>

41. <u>Carrot Family</u>

a. carrot

b. celery

c. parsnip

d. parsley

e. dill

f. fennel

g. anise

h. caraway

i. angelica

42. **Ginseng**

43. **Blueberry Family**

a. blueberry

b. cranberry

c. wintergreen

44. **Persimmon**

45. **Chicle**

46. **Tomato Family**

a. tomato

b. potato

c. eggplant

d. tobacco

47. **Peppermint Family**

a. peppermint

b. spearmint

c. horsemint

d. water mint

e. basil

f. lavender oil

g. rosemary

h. marjoram

i. sage

j. horehound

k. savory

l. thyme

m. Chinese artichoke

48. **Sweet Potato**

49. **Coffee**

50. **Elderberry**

51. **Melon Family**

a. melon

b. pumpkin

c. squash

d. cucumber

e. pickle

52. **Lettuce Family**

a. lettuce

b. endive

c. chicory

d. common artichoke

e. Jerusalem artichoke

f. sunflower

g. dandelion

h. chamomile

i. goldenrod

j. safflower

1. **Mollusks**

   A. **Subfamily: Pelecypods:**
      a. clam
      b. oyster
      c. mussel
      d. scallop
      e. cockle

   B. **Subfamily: Gastropods:**
      a. snail
      b. conch
      c. abalone

   C. **Subfamily: Cephalopods**

      a. squid
      b. octopus

2. **Crustacea**
   a. shrimp
   b. lobster
   c. crayfish
   d. crab

3. **Fish***

4. **Amphibia**
   Frog

5. **Reptiles**
   a. turtle
   b. snake
   c. alligator

6. **Birds**
   a. duck
   b. goose
   c. grouse
   d. prairie chicken
   e. quail
   f. peafowl
   g. domestic pheasant

h. domestic chicken
i. guinea fowl
j. turkey
k. pigeon

7. **<u>Mammals</u>**

a. opossum
b. rabbit
c. domestic guinea pig
d. muskrat
e. squirrel*
f. woodchuck
g. prairie dog
h. beaver
i. whale*
j. dolphin
k. porpoise
l. wolf
m. bear*
n. raccoon
o. lion
p. tiger
q. sea lion
r. walrus
s. seal
t. elephant
u. horse
v. pig
w. hippopotamus
x. camel
y. llama
z. deer
aa. elk
bb. moose
cc. caribou and reindeer
dd. giraffe
ee. antelope
ff. domestic cattle
gg. bison
hh. water buffalo
ii. African buffalo
jj. sheep
kk. goat

*All varieties

Appendix 4

HOW TO DEAL WITH YOUR YEAST/ MOLHYPERSENSITIVITY

I. <u>These foods may contain the yeast/mold group and should be avoided:</u>
   A. <u>YEAST FORM:</u>
      1. Baker's yeast (leavening):
         Bread and other yeast-containing pastries that "rise" on baking
      2. Brewers' yeast
         a. Alcoholic beverages of all types (beer, wine, whiskey, etc.)
         b. Vinegar of all types and any products containing vinegar READ LABELS!
      3. Miscellaneous:
         a. Sauerkraut, pickles, olives, all fermented and/or pickled prod-ucts, and fermented soy sauce
         b. Cured and pickled meat and fish

B. MYCELIAL FORM (Fluffy, cottony forms of mold)
All fermented cheeses (there are cheeses that are not fermented, such as: cream cheese, cottage cheese, ricotta, and yoghurt—which is a product of bacterial fermentation and not yeast fermentation)

C. MISCELLANEOUS:
Mushrooms, truffles

II. <u>These foods do not contain the yeast/ mold group and are acceptable:</u>

A. <u>Baked goods made without yeast leavening (baking powder leavening is acceptable—the kind without aluminum)</u>, matzo, and rice cakes. (Some patients react to baked goods, perhaps because of the gas oven in which they are baked.)

B. Fresh meats and fish and poultry

C. Fresh fruits and vegetables

©1989 Alfred V. Zamm, M.D.

Dear Reader,

Another Book in the Dr. Zamm's Medical Mysteries Series that you or somebody you know may find useful Additionally, from time to time you may wish to check with your bookseller for new additions to the Dr. Zamm's Medical Mysteries Series

AN ACTUAL CURE
ACID REFLUX
GERD

(Gastroesophageal Reflux Disease)

A Manganese
Nutritional Deficiency

Diet is NOT a Factor

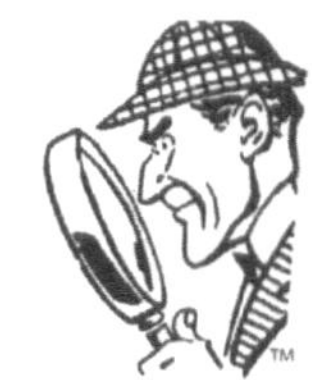

Who gets cured
Who doesn't
and why

Alfred V. Zamm, M.D.

DR. ZAMM'S MEDICAL MYSTERIES—VOL. 1 ED. 3

MACULAR DEGENERATION A SOLUTION

(Age-related Macular Degeneration—AMD)

A Taurine Nutritional Amino Acid Deficiency

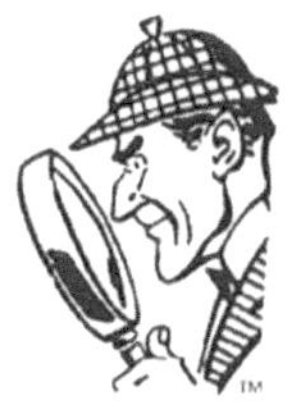

The patient had macular degeneration and was discovered to be deficient in the nutrient amino acid taurine.

He was given taurine:

1. His poor eyesight symptoms successfully improved.

2. The destructive progression of macular degeneration stopped.

Alfred V. Zamm, M.D.

DR. ZAMM'S MEDICAL MYSTERIES—VOL. 2 ED. 2

SECOND EDITION—ESSENTIAL NEW MATERIAL
LARGER TYPE

KIDNEY FAILURE A SOLUTION

(Dialysis became unnecessary)

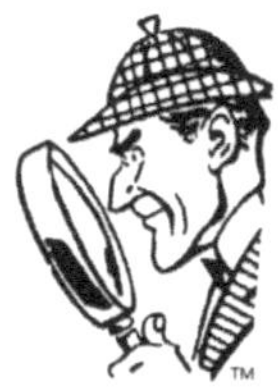

The patient was found to have food allergies
that were targeting her kidneys.

The responsible foods were removed from her diet.

Her abnormal kidney laboratory tests became normal

How this was done is explained in this step-by-step guidance manual.
Contains a treasure trove of scientific references

Alfred V. Zamm, M.D.

DR. ZAMM'S MEDICAL MYSTERIES SERIES—VOL. 3

Medical Secrets I Never Told You

(More Medical Mysteries by Dr. Zamm)

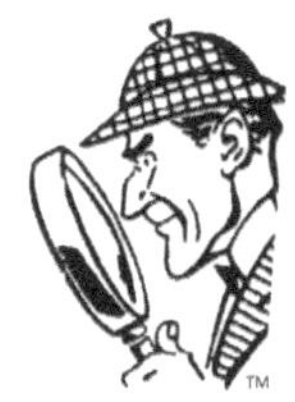

A COLLECTION OF
SURPRISING MEDICAL REVELATIONS
YOU NEED—BUT DIDN'T KNOW TO ASK

Alfred v. Zamm, M.D.

DR. ZAMM'S MEDICAL MYSTERIES SERIES—VOL. 4

COVID
AND
OTHER VIRAL CRIMINALS

How I Saved
My Grandson

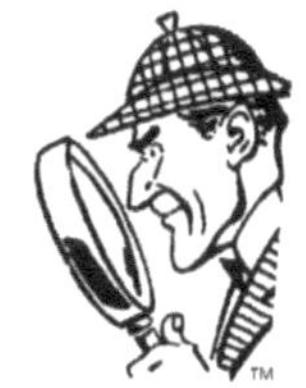

A Step-By-Step Explanation
of How I Did It
and
What You Need to Know

Alfred V. Zamm, M.D.

DR. ZAMM'S MEDICAL MYSTERIES SERIES—VOL. 5

MIGRAINE HEADACHES

I used to have them

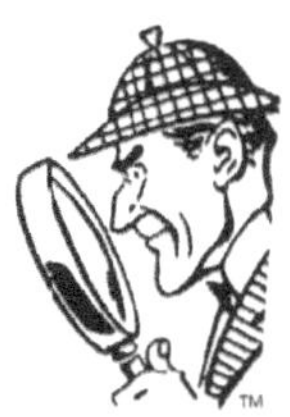

How I cured my headaches
A step-by-step explanation

Alfred V. Zamm, M.D.

DR. ZAMM'S MEDICAL MYSTERIES SERIES—VOL. 6

ACNE
AN ACTUAL
CURE

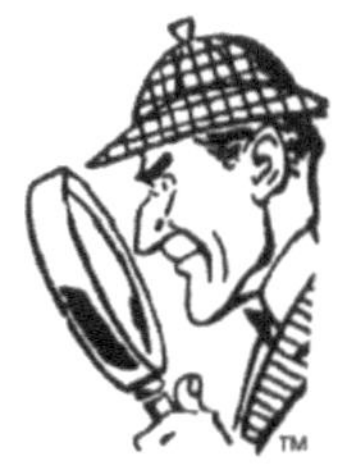

Who gets cured
Who doesn't
and why

Alfred V. Zamm, M.D.

DR. ZAMM'S MEDICAL MYSTERIES SERIES—VOL. 7 ED. 1